RELIEF FROM BACK PAIN
The Tollison Program

RELIEF FROM BACK PAIN

The Tollison Program

By C. DAVID TOLLISON, Ph.D.

President, Pain Therapy Centers™

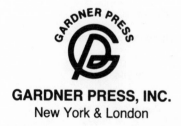

GARDNER PRESS, INC.
New York & London

Gardner Press, Inc.
19 Union Square West
New York, NY 10003

All foreign orders except Canada and South America to:
Afterhurst Limited
Chancery House
319 City Road
London N1, United Kingdom

Library of Congress Cataloging in Publication Data

PAIN THERAPY CENTERS is a registered trademark. All rights owned by Greenville Health Corporation.

Art by Bonnie Adamson
Photography by Alan Francis

This book is designed to provide advice and encouragement in the treatment and prevention of back pain. It is sold with the understanding that the publisher is not engaged in rendering medical service. If medical assistance or other professional advice is required, the services of a professional should be sought. No one should try any of the exercises or advice in this book without first consulting a physician.

Printed in the United States of America

Library of Congress Cataloging-in-Publication Data

Tollison, C. David.
  Relief from back pain, the Tollison program.

  Includes index.
  1. Backache. 2. Backache—Prevention. I. Title.
RD768.T65 1987   617′.56   86-26993
ISBN 0-89876-140-9

Book Design by Sidney Solomon

To Linda, Courtney, and David

CONTENTS

ACKNOWLEDGMENTS

Appreciation is extended to Gardner M. Spungin; Maggie Lattimore, for her tireless assistance in typing this manuscript and her countless hours of volunteer work to the community; the staff of PAIN THERAPY CENTERS; Melinda Davis, who accepts without hesitation the monumental task of keeping me organized; Jack A. Skarupa, president, Greenville Hospital System; Thomas E. Hassett, III, vice-president, Greenville Hospital System; Charles C. Boone, president, Spartanburg Reginal Medical Center; Kester S. Freeman, executive vice-president, Richland Memorial Hospital; Stephen H. Minsky, vice-president, Richland Memorial Hospital; John McGinnis, president, Bruce Hospital; H. Arnold Green, vice-president, Bruce Hospital; C. Glenn Trent, M.D.; John R. Satterthwaite, M.D.; Dr. and Mrs. Jerry C. Langley and family; Dr. and Mrs. Joseph W. Tollison and family; Mr. and Mrs. Walter E. Hayden; Mr. and Mrs. Fred L. Surett; Mrs. Wade A. Tollison; and Happi.

1

"OH, MY ACHING BACK!"

"Oh, my aching back!" How many times have you heard it said? How often have you felt that deep radiating ache? How many doctors have you visited in hope of pain relief? How long have you struggled with the frustration and anger that build as a result of unrelenting back pain? How frequently have you wished or heard it said that there should be something somewhere to ease the constant misery of back pain?

Over 50 million Americans suffer from backache. The long list includes such noted personalities as former President John Kennedy, golfers Lee Trevino and Fuzzy Zoeller, former Yankee shortstop Tony Kubek, football great Buddy Dial, hockey star Stan Mikita, politicians Edmund Muskie and Cyrus Vance, and entertainers Jerry Lewis, Joan Sutherland, and Barbra Streisand. And there are over eight million new victims each year.

Chronic back pain is increasingly recognized as a major personal, social, emotional, economic, and vocational disruption in the quality of our lives. In fact, in terms of numbers of victims and annual related costs, back pain ranks as our nation's third greatest health problem, behind heart disease and cancer.

My back feels like a bunch of hot pokers or arrows have been shoved into my spine. I can feel the heat and at times the pain is so severe that I almost think I can smell my flesh burning deep inside my back. Every moment sends a wave of blistering agony through my body like a giant fireworks display. My spine feels like it is on fire and there is no relief. I can't think or concentrate on anything except the horrible pain. I try to shift my concentration to conversation, people, television, or anything, but my attention always is pulled back to my agony. This has been going on now for almost three years and I don't know how much longer I can hold out. I feel like my body has been invaded by some kind of force determined to destroy me. It sounds crazy but I can almost close my eyes and picture an enemy in my back with those damn hot pokers sending waves of pain and nausea through me and I am helpless to resist. I've lost my wife and children and my job and almost everything else I've ever had. But I can't blame my family. I am living in pure hell and giving hell to everybody around me. I can't live like this much longer. I can't.

This is how William a 42 year-old former salesman, husband, father of two children, and community leader, described his crippling back pain to our staff at the PAIN THERAPY CENTER of Spartanburg, SC. He had been evaluated and treated by numerous orthopedic surgeons, neurologists, anesthesiologists, neurosurgeons, and internists. He had submitted to four back surgeries with the hope of finding relief that never came. By the time he was referred to PAIN THERAPY CENTERS℠, William had taken practically every available narcotic and nonnarcotic drug known and was abusing both medication and alcohol in an effort to escape the agony of his pain. He was seriously depressed and very near suicide.

THE ESCALATING NEMESIS OF BACK PAIN

More than 40 million Americans, will visit physicians this year with complaints of back pain.

While this in itself is a shocking statistic, consider that approximately 15 percent of back pain victims do not improve with either sophisticated medical treatment, including surgery, or the passage of time. Rather than enjoying eventual relief, many of these victims go from bad to worse and suffer increasingly severe pain and disability, despite the best efforts of modern medical science. Approximately 75 million Americans suffer chronic, handicapping pain, and a large percentage of these victims are plagued with backache. These individuals have typically suffered through several years of back agony, undergone two or more failed surgeries, are restricted in their jobs if not totally unable to work, take various and multiple medications for pain, experience chronic sleep disturbance, and are physically and psychologically strained and drained.

Surprised? Many people are since back pain seems such an innocuous problem to those fortunate individuals with good, strong, healthy backs. In this era of rampant heart disease, coronary bypass surgery, organ transplants, cancer, leukemia, and other dreaded diseases and life-saving interventions, the problem and treatment of back pain simply fails to impress those who have never known the agony of spinal discomfort. As a nation we have been conditioned to fear only the worst, the life-threatening, and the dramatic, and so we jog, exercise, quit smoking, attend stress innoculation workshops, and make every effort to avoid those diseases that endanger our lives.

And backache? It goes without saying that back pain generally poses no major direct threat to our longevity, nor does it draw enough national attention to warrant even a storyline in an episode of one of the many television medical shows. But while we are fast gaining a healthy respect for and knowledge of those issues and problems that affect the quantity of life, what steps are we taking to ensure the quality of our existence?

We as a nation are particularly illiterate in the management of one of the most costly, frequent, and painful disorders plaguing the quality of life. It is true that no one dies from benign backache, but many victims, like William, suffer a disabled and pleasureless existence. In addition, an alarming percentage of severely afflicted chronic back pain patients have no interest in longevity, but await death and its end to suffering with anticipation.

Perhaps a truly meaningful and enjoyable life cannot be measured only in terms of longevity. We have only to consider the chronic back pain victim whose every movement produces disabling pain to know that life must be a careful balance between quantity and quality. While heart disease, hypertension, cancer, leukemia, and other well-known problems certainly interrupt the quantity of life, back pain is gaining recognition as a major social, personal, industrial, and economic disruption in the quality of life. No matter how familiar I may be with these statistics and overall distress of chronic back pain, the reality of chronic discomfort never fails to impress me. Although back pain ranks as our nation's third greatest health problem, we do not organize ourselves in national and community associations to raise money for education, research, and support in the battle against it as we do to fight heart disease and cancer. Do our political and health leaders sound the alarm to fight chronic back pain? Do we pass legislation requiring manufacturers to place warnings on heavy boxes indicating proper lifting techniques to prevent back injuries the way cigarette manufacturers are required to warn the public against the potential dangers of smoking?

Unfortunately the answer is no. Ask the average person on the street about chronic pain and he or she is likely to have nothing to say. Ask the same person about alcoholism and you will probably hear about the very serious effects of this disease. Yet the annual expenditure on chronic pain is estimated at $60 billion whereas the expenditure on alcoholism, a far more publicized disease, is estimated at approximately $27 billion. Many of us who work in the field of chronic pain share with our patients a sense of mounting frustration over the national inattention and ignorance of one of its most costly, disrupting, and distressing health problems—*back pain!*

PAIN THERAPY CENTERS

PAIN THERAPY CENTERS℠, with locations in association with participating hospitals in numerous cities, was organized to help people who suffer intractable pain that has not been alleviated despite the best efforts of traditional medical care. Based on the initial limited success of some of the earliest so-called "pain clinics," we believed that treatment techiques, both old and new, could be refined, altered, and improved. We further believed that there was a better way to help pain sufferers than multiple surgeries, drug dependence, costly and lengthy psychotherapy, and disability. By borrowing treatment techniques that had been around for years and developing new approaches based on trial and error, we formulated a treatment program to view chronic pain not as a symptom of some underlying medical problem, but as a disease process itself.

Thousands of pain victims have now been treated in programs offered by our various centers. They have come from all walks of life and suffering a variety of pain problems. The key to our recognition and success lies in the development of an interdisciplinary staff specifically trained in both the physical and psychological rehabilitation of individuals in pain and our philosophy that chronic pain is a disease process in itself, that it is a disability to be overcome rather than a problem to be cured, and that chronic pain victims suffer one of the least understood and multifaceted health problems known. Pain patients want to improve and, with proper treatment and education, can return to a more normal and productive life-style. We know this from experience.

We do not perform magic or miracles. But a large number of our patients report a significant decrease in their pain, and even more tell us that they are managing their discomfort better without the disruption to their lives and relationships that was prevailent before treatment. Victims who come to our centers addicted to multiple medications for pain control leave drug-free and effectively controlling their pain. Many individuals who have been disabled from work are able to return to employment and a more stable financial situation. And then there are those who leave us with an assessment similar to that reported by a middle-aged former truck driver treated at our Pain Therapy Center of Columbia: "For the first time in over five years, I've got this pain problem under control. Now I tell my pain what I'm going to do, rather than the pain telling me what I'm going to do." Considering the condition that many of our patients are in when they come to us, perhaps this is as close to a miracle as we will ever see! As founder and director of Pain Therapy Centers, I have learned to combat pain and suffering on a daily basis and to consider every patient's success a miracle.

THE BACK: A HISTORY OF ABUSE AND MISUSE

I frequently tell my patients that when Eve offered the apple to Adam, a major and everlasting mistake was made prior to the well-known error of taking a big bite. What was this monumental mistake? Adam *stood* up to accept it!

Part of the reason that humans experience the agony of back pain is our insistence on standing erect. Ever since we assumed an upright position, the lower back has suffered.

Humans do not have the structural advantage of walking on all fours, with the pelvis tilted forward and our body weight evenly distributed. Instead humans walk upright, with the lower back bearing the brunt of the body's weight. In addition, the lower back has inherited the ever-increasing stress of daily living, poor posture, lack of exercise, and overeating. Back pain may have started with our ancestors taking that first step on two legs and this "advance-ment" has plagued us ever since.

Back pain victims can learn a great deal from our four-legged friends. An aching back feels much improved when you are on all fours. This is so because your body weight is evenly distributed over a greater area and the pelvis is tilted forward in a neutral position. Low back pressure, weight, stress, and *pain* are reduced. In fact, this technique for pain relief works so well that in Chapter 14 you will find a series of back exercises and illustrations of proper body mechanics called the "pelvic tilt." We teach this technique to our back pain patients in our programs and it often provides a meas-ure of relief.

THE BAD HABIT OF PAIN

"Hurting" can become a habit. As odd as it might sound, psy-chologists have known for years that any human, under the proper circumstances, can develop a "pain habit." And make no mistake about it—pain that is suffered because of a pain habit is just as discomforting as the agony experienced when a finger is crushed by an automobile door.

Perhaps the simplest illustration of pain as a bad habit is the phenomenon termed "phantom limb pain." Phantom limb pain is a fairly common complaint reported by individuals who have under-gone the surgical amputation of one or more limbs. Occasionally these individuals will suffer pain in a particular limb for some time before the decision is made to amputate. Following surgery, the patient continues to report pain in the limb although the arm or leg is no longer attached to the body. Could it be that the victim suffers for so long that a habit of pain is established that is so strongly ingrained in the subconscious that pain messages continue even after the painful limb is removed? Although some researchers argue that the phenomenon of phantom limb pain is a bit more compli-cated than described, many scientists strongly support the theory of a pain habit.

Before considering other examples of how pain can become a bad habit, let us look for a moment at how we are socialized or conditioned to perceive pain. When you were a child riding your bicycle and fell and scraped your elbow, how did your mother and father react? Consider the following and what each response would tell you about pain.

"Oh baby, I'm sorry! Here, let me carry you inside and get some medicine and a bandaid and I'll take care of you. Then I'll get you a good cold drink and I'll read you a story."

"Oh baby, I'm sorry! Come here and let me see how badly you are hurt. I don't think you should try and ride that bicycle any more because you might get hurt again."

"Oh, you had an accident, didn't you? You'll be okay, it's just a scrape. Get back on your bike and show me how you've been practicing."

If your parents responded as in our first example fairly consistently, you might grow to associate pain with needing time away from activity to refresh, rest, and recover. If you later suffered back pain as an adult, is it possible that by habit you began thinking of going to see a doctor, just to get it "checked out," and maybe taking some time off from work to rest and recover?

If the reaction in our second example was fairly common, you might learn to associate certain activities with the *expectancy* of pain. If you later suffered a painful back injury at work, is it possible that your disability was prolonged because you have a conditioned habit to expect pain if you return to the same activity?

The response in our third example could foster the most appropriate and healthiest perception of pain. If you later suffered a painful back injury, you might continue your life-style as best you could until the pain subsided.

These are just three examples of how patterns of child socialization can influence our perception of pain and cause us to develop habits of pain. There are many others.

For example, suppose that you suffered a very painful back injury that forced you to bed for several weeks. Let us further assume that your previously inattentive spouse, children, neighbors, and friends suddenly paid you a great deal of attention. Everyone visited you daily, brought you food and snacks, took care of your yard work and other responsibilities, and repeatedly encouraged you to take it easy.

If the above illustration were true, how rapidly would you be inclined to recover? It is possible that the positive reinforcement for hurting might subconsciously motivate you to continue hurting. A friend told me that as a teenager he was once hospitalized for treatment of injuries sustained in an automobile accident. His primary problem at the time was a painful, although not serious, neck injury.

Part of his treatment included twice-daily physical therapy, which included soothing massages administered by a young, attractive therapist. Years later he would periodically experience episodes of neck pain that would be relieved if his wife massaged his neck. He attributed these painful episodes to the lingering effects of his earlier injury.

My friend, who is now a practicing psychiatrist, finally hit upon the fact that he seemed to develop his periodic episodes of adult neck pain when he felt insecure, vulnerable, threatened, and in need of love and affection. His wife's simple massage was not a cure, but her attention and gentle touch did wonders! Upon further introspection he recalled the events of years before and the attractive therapist who calmed his fears and pain with her consideration and soft touch. With this realization his episodes of neck pain were eliminated and my friend became a believer in the power of psychological reinforcement.

A final example of pain habits is the important role of avoidance. Want to avoid work? "I've got a backache." Want to avoid school? "I've got a tummyache." Want to avoid sex? "I've got a headache." No doubt most of us learned as children the effective use of physical complaints to avoid unpleasant situations or activities.

Let us suppose that you are tired of your husband leaving the family every weekend to play golf or go fishing. Occasional weekends or even alternate weekends are fine, but never missing a weekend for years and years is just too much! One Friday you develop a very uncomfortable aching in your lower back and you go to bed to rest. Guess what happens the next morning? For the first time in years, your aching back has accomplished what hours of discussing, reasoning, and pleading had never come close to accomplishing. Your husband cancels his weekend golfing trip! Your aching back is to thank for allowing you to avoid a most unpleasant situation. Although your back is quite discomforting, can you see the potential for another subconscious episode of back pain the next time you feel you have taken all of the neglect you can stand?

DO YOU REALLY WANT TO GET BETTER?

However unbelievable it may seem, some back pain victims do not really want to rid themselves of pain. For these individuals the cost of living a pain-free existence is just too high.

Consider a less educated, nonskilled employee fighting to scratch out a living. Twenty years ago appropriate jobs were plentiful and competition in the job market was minimal. But also consider the explosion of technological sophistication that has taken place in the past 20 years. Skilled artisans have proliferated and competition has increased. Jobs are more complex and require greater training and skill. Our unskilled friend knows that his job security is becoming increasingly threatened. He fears he will lose his job and be unable to find another. He worries that he may lose the very few material things he has managed to secure and wonders how he will provide for his family.

One day he trips over some boxes at work and strains his back. The company doctor assures him that he can return to work in two weeks and sends him home to recover. Two weeks later he is not improved so he is excused from work for four additional weeks. His worker's compensation checks arrive each week and he is being paid to stay home and avoid the steadily increasing stress related to his job. Months pass and he files for Social Security Disability due to his "horrible back pain." He is turned down for disability so he files an appeal and hurts more than ever.

It is unfortunate that our system of worker's compensation, disability, and litigation is based on the victim's success in having a problem that our health care system can't resolve. Of course, on a conscious level, few people would ever accept pain for money. In fact, most pain victims would gladly sacrifice any financial gain for even a brief reprieve from their agonizing discomfort. But the subconscious mind may not be thinking on the same rational and logical level that characterizes the conscious mind. Perhaps the subconscious mind considers that continued pain is the only way out of a financial bind, the only solution to threatened job security, or the only means to have security needs met. In support of this notion, a number of research articles report that back pain victims with pending litigation do not enjoy the improvement in their conditions that nonlitigation back pain victims enjoy, until the litigation is settled! After settlement, there is little difference in the improvement shown by the two groups.

Do you have a need to hurt? Consciously the answer is probably no, but how about at the subconscious level? Examine the various aspects of your life. Are there reinforcements for hurting, opportunities for avoidance, or patterns of childhood conditioning and socialization that might play a role in your back discomfort? Be honest in your examination. There is no shame in being the victim of subconscious conditioning.

NO PAIN PROBLEM IS HOPELESS AND NO VICTIM IS HELPLESS

It disturbs me to hear a pain victim told to "go home and live with it, nothing more can be done." Isn't that another way of saying, "Give up, quit trying, it's hopeless?"

The vast majority of patients treated in our programs suffer the complicating factor of depression, in addition to their pain problem. And little wonder—most of our patients have been told to give up the fight because pain relief is hopeless.

Hopelessness is very closely related to helplessness, which has been identified as one of the leading causes of depression. Dealing with unrelenting pain and being told that there is nothing that can be done is a prime example of perpetuating pain victims' feelings of helplessness.

Dr. Martin E. P. Seligman, from the University of Pennsylvania, conducted a series of important studies concerning "learned helplessness." Dr. Seligman used an enclosed chamber, called a shuttle box, which has a small hurdle in the middle that separates the chamber into two compartments. As a rule, if a dog is placed in one compartment and the floor of the compartment is wired to deliver a series of electric shocks, the dog quickly learns to jump the hurdle to the other side, which is shock-free. In a short time, the dog will learn to jump from side to side to avoid the shocks.

Dr. Seligman then altered the usual procedure by placing dogs in a harness that allowed no escape, and then delivered a series of electric shocks. Initially the dogs howled, became agitated, and tried desperately to escape the pain. But eventually the dogs simply "gave up" even trying to avoid the shocks, becoming passive.

The next step was to remove the harness again and place the dogs back into the shuttle box. Although the opportunity to escape the pain of the shocks now existed, the dogs sat passively, resigned to their fate. The dogs had *learned to become helpless* and had given up hope of relief. A possibility for relief was present, but the dogs had become too helpless to take advantage of it.

Does this sound familiar? Can you see how being told to simply "live" with your pain and quit trying or hoping for relief could easily lead to a state of learned helplessness? I am convinced that the research of Dr. Seligman has important implications for chronic back pain victims.

If you are a victim of chronic back pain, I hope you will never accept the idea that "there is no hope." I hope also that you will not neglect your life, responsibilities, and pleasures in an obsessive, desperate, and prolonged search for relief. A proper balance in life is critically important and it is imperative that you maintain your hope *while* you attend to your responsibilities. To neglect either disrupts the balance and may well spell defeat.

By the same token, I am not suggesting that you submit to potentially dangerous and harmful "treatments." Finding someone to operate on a painful back or give you drugs to ease the pain is not a difficult task. If one or two doctors told you that surgery would not help and suddenly a new doctor is anxious to operate, get another opinion before agreeing. If you are taking medication but continue to suffer and a doctor increases the strength of your drug or adds a second and third medication, be careful. The typical patient treated in our PAIN THERAPY CENTERS℠ programs has undergone an average of three unsuccessful surgeries for pain relief and many are addicted to or are abusing medications. Maintain your hope for relief, but utilize caution and intelligence in your search.

If conventional medical science offers you no further hope for back pain relief, consider the unconventional. Pain has plagued human beings since long before our age of modern miracle medicine and our ancestors may not have been as simple and limited as we often believe. Many treatment techniques considered outdated by "sophisticated science" are being reevaluated and rediscovered as useful in the management of pain. Hypnosis, acupuncture, yoga, attitude, electrical therapies, an overlooked food substance called tryptophan, or any of the many other treatment techniques described in this book may provide victims with a measure of pain relief.

No pain problem is hopeless, at least as long as you don't give up. If you feel you have tried everything but continue in pain, maybe what you need is a "game plan" for relief.

A GAME PLAN FOR RELIEF

How many times have you listened to coaches in postgame interviews explain their team's loss with the phrase, "We just got away from our game plan." A game plan sounds simple enough—an organized, planned, and charted course leading to a goal—but getting away from the plan can result in complexity and frustration.

If you have visited numerous doctors and undergone a variety of tests and treatments without success, perhaps you need to develop an organized, planned, and charted course leading to your goal of back pain relief!

Let us start with attitude. If you are to win the fight against back pain, you must first develop a winning attitude. Too many chronic pain victims expect each new treatment to fail. It is easy to understand how this negative attitude develops when one is subjected to multiple treatments without success. But consider that a negative attitude may prolong your misery. At our PAIN THERAPY CENTERS℠, we invite patients who have graduated from our treatment program to return to talk to those undergoing treatment. Seeing a "successful graduate" gives other sufferers hope and convinces them that chronic back pain can be conquered. It helps develop in our current patients the same winning attitude that helped our graduates learn to control pain effectively. Since you have come this far in reading this book without tossing it aside in disbelief, you still have a bit of a winning attitude and are willing to give pain control another try.

The second part of developing a game plan for pain relief is motivation. This book is a self-help text. There is very little information in it that will make a measurable difference in reducing your pain without your practice and application.

Notice that I said *your* practice and application. Whether or not the techniques described are worth the cost of the book or the time it takes to read is largely dependent on you. I tell our patients that they will get out of our treatment program exactly what they put into it. Whether you will benefit from this program of pain control is a prediction I cannot make with total certainty. But there is one guarantee. If you are not motivated enough to assume the responsibility for applying and practicing the techniques described, they will certainly provide no relief! The decision is yours.

The final part of developing a game plan for pain relief is a commitment on your part to become a student of the back. The more you learn about the back, the more you will be able to compensate for your weaknesses, understand your problem, and take the necessary steps to control your pain. The program for pain relief outlined here is divided into three major sections: (1) understanding back pain, (2) evaluation of back pain, and (3) treatment of back pain. Each section is critically important in the overall relief program. I urge you to read the entire book through twice before beginning the pain relief program. The information presented is necessary for successful pain control.

Now that we have developed a game plan for pain relief, we are ready to begin. The referee's whistle has sounded and the contest is under way. Are you ready? If so, let us begin with a thorough understanding of pain and the spine and build toward pain relief!

2

A PAINLESS COURSE IN SPINAL ANATOMY

The anatomy of the back should be of more than merely academic interest. How the back is constructed and how it works should be of concern to all those who experience back problems, as well as those who want to prevent them. Understanding the basic composition and mechanics of the spine allows us to create techniques to relieve discomfort and to prevent spinal overload and injury. But we shy away from studying the back as if this mysterious part of our anatomy were too complex for the average pain sufferer to understand. Those few who undertake to learn are often surprised to discover that while a thorough understanding of the spine can represent a complex endeavor, the basic functioning of the back is really quite simple. In fact, anyone with an elementary understanding of levers, pulleys, and weights, or even anyone who has ever played with a child's seesaw, can easily understand the basics of the back. But do doctors and back pain victims take the time to talk, explain, study, and understand the back? Too often, the answer is no!

Even victims who have suffered years of backache and have undergone numerous tests and surgeries have almost no knowledge of the back. Though most do not understand the cause of their back pain, if asked, the majority will quickly parrot a traditional medical textbook explanation complete with terminology and medical jargon that would impress even the most scholarly medical school professor. But it is very unusual that the patient actually comprehends the explanation.

Yet these same people have trusted their medical and surgical care, and even their very lives, to a physician who is usually a stranger. I cannot help but wonder how many of these patients would consider dropping off their automobiles to an unknown mechanic with the order, "No need to explain the problem to me, just repair it!" I suspect very few.

So let us spend a few minutes learning the basic composition of the human spine. Education is an important part of the Tollison program and PAIN THERAPY CENTERS℠ treatment program.

THE PARTS OF THE SPINE

Your back is working 24 hours a day, every day of the year. Every time you lift, sit, stand, or even lie down you are using your back. And consider the abuse that the back endures—sports, obesity, improper lifting, physically deconditioned life-styles, pregnancies, poor posture, accidents, anxiety, tension, and more. When my patients ask, "Why do I have to have this backache?" I respond, "All things considered, the fact that you suffer back pain is probably more normal than abnormal." Recognizing the composition of the back and the abuse that most of us impose upon the spine, the fact that back pain is our nation's third most frequent health care complaint is hardly surprising. Let us see why.

Vertebrae

Supporting the back is the spinal column, made up of bony vertebrae. From the base of your skull to the bottom of your tailbone, you have 33 or 34 vertebrae. There are numerous problems that can develop at every level of the column, although some regions are more susceptible than others.

The vertebrae are divided into five major regions of the spine—cervical, thoracic, lumbar, sacrum, and coccyx (Figure 2-1). The cervical, thoracic, and lumbar regions are flexible and have a total of 24 vertebrae among them. The sacrum and coccyx regions are two fused regions with nine or ten bones.

The neck or *cervical* region has seven vertebrae. These vertebrae are the smallest in the spine and are particularly susceptible to "whiplash" injuries from automobile crashes or other accidents.

The midback or *thoracic* region has 12 vertebrae. These are the least frequently injured or damaged vertebrae in the spine, generally due to the position of the thoracic verebrae and the decreased amount of stress and pressure on this region. The thoracic vertebrae are attached to the ribs and provide strong spinal support and stabilization.

The largest vertebrae in the spine are the five *lumbar* vertebrae, the most frequently injured vertebrae in the spine because of the position of the lower back in the body and the resulting pressure and stress on the region. Most herniated or "ruptured" disks develop in the area of the lumbar spine, which is also the area where most spinal surgeries are performed.

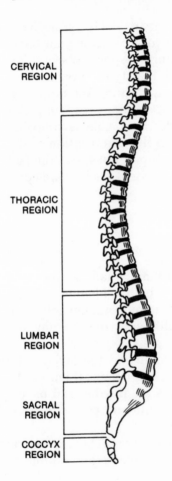

CERVICAL
REGION

THORACIC
REGION

LUMBAR
REGION

SACRAL
REGION

COCCYX
REGION

Figure 2-1—The vertebrae are divided into five major regions of the spine—cervical, thoracic, lumbar, sacrum, and coccyx.

During the formative months before birth, our *sacrum* region is actually five separate bones. But by the time we are born, the sacrum has fused into one immobile and solid bone. The sacral region is not a common trouble spot for most back pain victims.

Finally, we have four or five small vertebral bones in the tailbone or *coccyx* region. As strange as it may seem, some people have four coccyx bones while others have five. According to evolutional theory, the coccyx is the only remnant left of a tail we inherited from the apes a few million years ago. The coccyx is most frequently injured during hard falls when the victims land in sitting positions.

To simplify matters, doctors and health professionals use the five identified regions of the spine to designate an area of vertebrae or disk trouble. For example, T10 is the tenth thoracic vertebra and L4-L5 is the disk that is between the fourth and fifth vertebrae.

Disks

Between the bony vertebrae of the spine lie the useful but sometimes troublesome disks. By separating and cushioning the vertebrae from each other, disks act as shock absorbers. In fact, in a healthy back the oval-shaped disks absorb pressure from any downward force on the spine and then "bounce back" to their original shape (Figure 2-2). Spinal disks are very tightly attached to the adjacent vertebrae above and below in a fashion that would make the manufacturers of "Super Glue" green with envy. This bond is so tight that a terrible accident, such as a severe fall or automobile accident, will break or crush the hard bony vertebrae before the adhesive bond is broken!

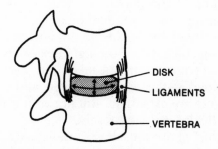

DISK

LIGAMENTS

VERTEBRA

Figure 2-2—Spinal disks are resilient and are therefore able to absorb pressure and return to their original shape.

If you were to examine a human spinal disk, you might be impressed with its similarity to a radial-belted automobile tire. Disks are protected by a tough, elastic shell made up of crisscrossed layers of fibers that strengthen and protect the disk. Another way to imagine a spinal disk is to consider a jelly donut (with a very tough outer covering). Inside the disk is a soft, jellylike substance. If you "rupture" or herniate a disk, it is this inner substance that "slips" out of the disk and frequently causes trouble.

While many people automatically associate severe back pain with a herniated or "ruptured" disk, this is usually not the cause. A very small percentage of back pain victims suffer herniated disks. There are numerous reasons for a back to hurt, and disk trouble represents but one of many. Many victims assume that "any back pain that hurts this badly must surely be a ruptured disk." The fact is that the intensity of pain does not generally suggest any particular cause of backache. I have seen patients with severe muscular strain suffer more agony than others with herniated disk. As we shall see in later chapters, the degree or intensity of pain is determined by numerous factors beyond the actual pathology or physical cause of back pain.

Muscles

Like the comedian Roger Dangerfield, our muscles "get no respect." In fact, not only are our muscles not given the respect due, but more often then not they are perceived in a negative manner. For example, we compliment someone when we say that the person is smart, "brainy," or has a big heart. But what about muscles? "All muscles, no brains,""muscle-bound," and "muscling in on us" hardly carry complimentary connotations.

Even the majority of physicians do not give muscles the respect they are due. When you have a thorough physical examination, your blood pressure and pulse rate are taken, an electrocardiogram is recorded, your blood and urine are analyzed, and your heart, lungs, nose, ears, and eyes are examined. But are your muscles examined for strength and flexibility? Very rarely.

The near-neglect of our muscles is unfortunate since they assist or are responsible for countless tasks. When we walk and talk, we use our muscles. When we work with our hands, such as writing, we use our muscles. And practically any movement of the body uses the muscles in the back. In addition, our muscles allow us to express ourselves to others around us. When we show our thoughts and feelings by facial movements, when we laugh, when we cry, and when we dance, we use our muscles. We use our muscles constantly to show what we think and feel, and can do. And this applies as much to the abstract thinker as it does to the laborer. The thinker or the laborer who is burdened with back pain and stiff, aching spinal muscles is soon limited in both performance and motivation.

The entire spine is supported by a magnificent and elaborate organization of muscles, the first line of defense against gravity and other outside forces. But in order to function correctly, and to offset sudden blows or continuous strain, the spine needs help. This help is given by the back and trunk muscles—and not only the back muscles, but stomach muscles and hip flexors and hip extensors as well. And few examples illustrate the concept of "teamwork" better than the spinal muscles.

The back muscles are numerous but small, with the exception of the large kiteshaped muscle called the trapezius, which starts at the base of the skull and fans out to the outer edges of the shoulders before pulling back to a point halfway down the center of the back. Because they are small, they must work in teams of two or three to get the job done. And the job of supporting and moving the body is a Herculean task indeed! Since the back muscles must work together, a weakness in any one muscle group can put excessive strain on another, which can upset your spine's balance. If the muscles fail to keep the joints of the back within their normal range of movement, ligaments are stretched and may be strained.

Muscles are very important to the health of the back and may well represent the single greatest cause of back pain. Stomach and leg muscles also play a critical role in back care. Weak stomach muscles can allow a "pot belly" to overload the spine and tilt the back out of balance. To compensate, back muscles must tighten and remain tight, which increases pain. Strong legs balance the body, including the spine. I frequently tell our patients that strong legs act to steady and support the back like training wheels on a bicycle.

Your muscles can be trained. If you take the trouble to train them properly through special exercise, they can become strong, relaxed, and an ally against back pain. On the other hand, they can become shortened, tense, and an aggravating factor in back pain as a result of lack of exercise and overirritation. In later chapters we will further clarify how the spinal muscles can result in enormous misery for back pain victims. More important, however, we will present a series of exercises and techniques developed at our centers that have proven useful in transforming a group of spasming, aching muscles into an aid in back pain relief.

Nerves

The human nervous system is a most complex communication network linking different parts of the body, as well as the body and the brain. And despite the advanced technology that characterizes modern computers and information systems, we have never designed a communication system that comes close to matching the sophistication of the human nervous system.

An easy way to consider the function of our nerves is to imagine the telephone communications system of a giant company with the switchboard located at the corporate headquarters and lines of communication going out to numerous branch offices. Without an elaborate system of communication, corporate headquarters has no idea of what is going on in the field and the branch office in Chicago does not know what the branch offices in Atlanta, Dallas, and Los Angeles are doing. Communication is the key, if the company is to function smoothly and effectively whole.

Our bodies are similar. For one's body to work smoothly and effectively as a whole, it must have a system of communication. Our nerves serve this important function.

The human spine is a body part particularly rich with nerve supply and there is a close relationship between back pain and the nerves in and around the spine (Figure 2-3). For example, in some instances, back pain can be caused by actual injury to one of the spinal nerves. In Chapter 4 we will discuss in greater detail the condition commonly referred to as "pinched nerve." In other cases the nerves in the back pick up the message of pain from some malfunctioning part of the back and communicate the pain signal to the brain.

The nerves of the spine are divided into the same regions as the vertebrae and, for order and simplicity, are given the same designations–C3, T5, L4, and so on. However, there is one minor variation. Because there are eight cervical nerves as compared with seven cerical vertebrae, the "C" or cervical series for nerves runs up to C8, while the C series for vertebrae stops at C7.

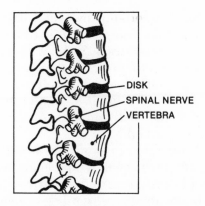

Figure 2-3—Back pain can result from an injury such
as "pinching" of one of the spinal nerves.

Nerve roots that exit the spinal column through small openings
made by the connection of two vertebrae are often involved in complaints of back pain (Figure 2-3). Nerve roots collect together to form
nerve branches that run from the spine to the various parts of the
body. For example, nerve roots from the lower lumbar and upper
sacral areas of the spine join together to form the sciatic nerve,
which runs down the back of the leg. This can sometimes cause you
to have pain in one or both legs as a result of damage in the lower
back. In fact, your lower back may feel fine while one or both legs
ache. The culprit is still the lower back, but try to explain that to
someone who experiences pain in only the left calf.

Spinal Cord

The human spinal cord can be thought of as the "expressway to
the brain." It is a delicate and sophisticated communication vehicle.
While countless numbers of nerves acting as receiving stations pick
up the message of pain and forward the impulse through a labyrinth
of twists, turns, detours, and junctions on the way to the spine, it
is the spinal cord that ultimately receives the pain impulse, refines
and modifies the message, and sends it speeding to the brain for
registration and decoding. This is important since it is the brain, not
the back, that tells us when we hurt. For example, if an individual
suffers damage to the spinal cord that results in paralysis from the
waist down (a condition known as paraplegia), he or she may have

no feeling in the legs. I have known several paraplegics who sustained serious burns to the legs from sitting too close to a fire, or suffered other serious leg injuries because, without clear pain transmission by the spinal cord to the brain, they were *unaware* of pain. In other words, if the brain does not receive the message of pain and appropriately register the impulse, for all intents and purposes we do not hurt and may be totally unaware of serious and mounting damage being done to our bodies.

The spinal cord is encased in a tough protective covering called the spinal column or spinal canal, which is located adjacent to the spinal vertebrae and disks (Figure 2-4). Rather than being just a messenger to the brain, the spinal cord performs many functions that for years were thought to be the exclusive role of the brain. When your doctor gives you the familiar reflex test by tapping your knee lightly with a rubber hammer, the nerve impulses race up your leg as far as the spinal cord, but no further. Your spinal cord responds to the impulses by ordering a muscular reaction and the lower leg jerks forward.

All along the spinal column are small openings between the bony projections or adjacent vertebrae. These openings allow an exit for pairs of spinal nerves branching out, right and left, from the spinal cord. Because of the position of the spinal column to the adjacent vertebrae and disk, any bulging or herniation of a disc can spell potential trouble for the spinal cord and the victim. As we shall see in Chapters 4 and 9, this is a situation that can result in miserable back and leg pain, or even neurologic damage.

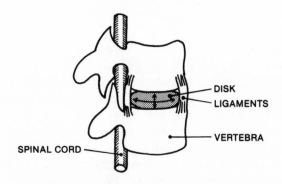

Figure 2-4—The delicate spinal cord is protected from injury by the spinal column.

HOW THE BACK WORKS

Think for a moment about the location of the back, particularly the lower back. If we divide the vertical adult into right and left halves, the center runs right along the spine through the lower back (Figure 2-5). Furthermore, if we divide this same adult into upper and lower halves along a horizontal plane, again the center crosses the body at the level of the lower back (Figure 2-5). With this idea in mind, and borrowing from the laws of physics, we can consider the lower back as serving a purpose similar to that of a fulcrum. You will recall that a fulcrum is the center point and area of particular pressure and strain along a plane.

A child's seesaw may better explain the tremendous demands placed on the spine and the vulnerability of this part of our anatomy.

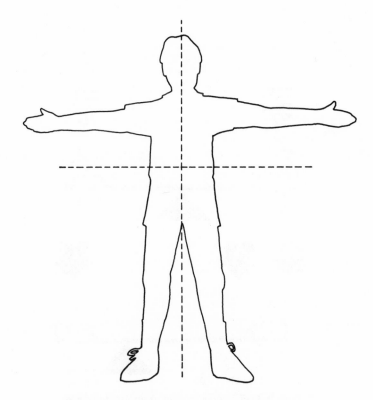

Figure 2-5—The horizontal and vertical axis of the body is located in the lower back.

As can be seen in Figure **2-7,** a seesaw ordinarily has a nearly equal weight distribution on either side of the fulcrum. With this distribution there is balance and smooth operation of the seesaw similar to the normal, trouble-free functioning of a balanced spine.

But what if we interfere with the balance of the seesaw? Let us suppose that we position the fulcrum so that there is twice the weight and pressure on one side of the center point (Figure 2-7). If this occurs, the child on the short side of the seesaw must exert twice as much downward thrust in order to maintain equilibrium and avoid tipping the balance. The child on the short side is now working against a ratio of two to one.

A similar situation occurs when we misuse, and abuse, our backs. The human spine was operationally designed and intended to be in perfect balance. But consider what happens when you lift a box or object with your arms straightened and extended before you. For

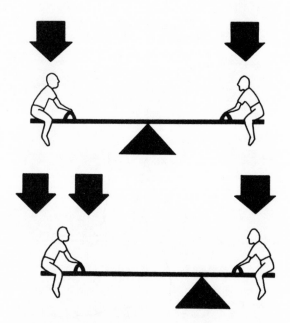

Figure 2-7—The child on the shorter side of the seesaw must exert twice as much downward thrust in order to maintain equilibrium.

the sake of example, let us assume that the distance from your midspine to fingertips is 30 inches, and the distance from your midspine to your back muscles is one inch. If this is the case, you are working at a 30 to one ratio. If you lift a ten-pound box, this ratio means you will have to provide 300 pounds of downward thrust on the back in order to keep the spine balanced and avoid tipping over! Since your back would have great difficulty providing that intensity of force, chances are good that your stomach muscles would be called on to assist. And if the weight to be lifted increased, other body parts would be enlisted to help the overworked and burdened spine.

In Chapters 10 and 14, we will look in more detail at how the back works and concentrate on outlining a number of useful techniques to reduce the enormous strain on our mechanical fulcrum. The lever or seesaw action of our spines can generate extreme spinal stress and strain, and can also be used to our advantage. The difference is in knowing how the back works and a few tricks for proper spinal care.

But first let us look at the biphasic nature of pain. A better understanding of this often neglected and misunderstood phenomenon will benefit our efforts to build a strong and effective arsenal to battle chronic back pain.

3

THE BIPHASIC NATURE OF PAIN

The word "pain" is derived from the Latin word *poena*, meaning "punishment," and both pain and punishment originate from the Sanskrit root *pu*, meaning "sacrifice." The idea of punishment and sacrifice of self in the experience of pain can be traced back to the first chapter of *Genesis* and even earlier in history to the *Upanishad*, one of the Holy Scriptures of Hinduism. For years pain and suffering were considered emotional phenomena of religious and philosophical study rather than an appropriate consideration for physicians. Aristotle (384–322 B.C.) expressed the common belief of his time when he defined pain as "a passion of the soul," an emotional outburst of the human heart. For over 2000 years the Aristotelian ideas about pain dominated, and people accepted pain and suffering as part of emotional and religious experience.

Not until the end of the nineteenth century did physiologic research open the door to the scientific and experimental investigation of pain. Then the pendulum quickly swung to the other extreme as an overly optimistic breed of scientists maintained that all pain problems could be solved by proper understanding and application of the mechanisms of physical laws.

Thus, at the beginning of the twentieth century, a great number of writings, including several literary classics, dealt with pain as a purely physical sensation with its own specific physical explanation and not a great deal different from the other five human senses. From this general perspective it was logically concluded that if pain is a physical phenomenon, it should be controlled by depressing pain receptors or blocking its pathways throughout the body.

Unfortunately the results of controlling chronic pain by surgical or chemical blocking of nerve pathways have been disappointing. Although medicine is generally able temporarily to abate the suffering from chronic diseases, it is not without consequences. Many patients go on to cope with what many consider to be an equal or even greater price, that of drug addiction or neurologic damage when nerve pathways are destroyed. As a result the explanation of pain as a purely biologic phenomenon has also lost support among most physicians who take the oldest rule of the medical profession seriously: "*primum non nocere*" (first, do no harm).

A quick perusal of the current literature on pain is certain to reveal the state of confusion surrounding theories that attempt to explain pain's course and mechanism. The pendulum is without question swinging again. The early Aristotelian concept of pain as a spiritual and emotional state is today considered an oversimplification, as is the later nineteenth century idea of pain as a specific biologic phenomenon. The modern health-care practitioner is confronted with increasing evidence that while there does exist a biologic network subserving the sensation of pain, the routine functioning of the network is greatly influenced by psychological or emotional factors in the form of stress and pressures, as well as the influence of learning processes. In fact, today pain is generally considered a complex *psychobiological* perception composed of at least two major components: *biology*, or physical, and *psychology*.

ACUTE VERSUS CHRONIC PAIN

Pain is a subjective experience; it is a personal possession, a private feeling, and as individual as a fingerprint. In general terms, there are two types of pain: acute and chronic. *Acute* pain is a message to its victim; *chronic* pain serves no identified useful purpose (Table 3-1).

Pulling the tangles out of your hair in the morning or a shaving razor "nick" of a facial blemish may cause some short-term acute pain. Slamming an automobile door on a finger or burning your hand on a hot oven may cause some longer lasting pain. You may twist your ankle walking across the yard and a hangnail may annoy you all day. And if you argue with your spouse or the children make excessive demands, a headache may be your reward at day's end.

Table 3-1
Comparison of Acute and Chronic Pain

ACUTE PAIN	CHRONIC PAIN
USEFUL	LITTLE SIGNIFICANCE
BRIEF DURATION	MORE THAN SIX MONTHS' DURATION
TREATMENT WELL DEFINED AND USUALLY SUCCESSFUL	TREATMENT MULTIFACTORIAL AND WITH LIMITED SUCCESS
DRUG THERAPY LIMITED WITH FEW COMPLICATIONS	DRUG THERAPY PROLONGED WITH MANY COMPLICATIONS
SYMPATHY APPROPRIATE	SYMPATHY MAY BE INAPPROPRIATE
NO PERMANENT DISABILITY	PERMANENT MANAGEMENT

Tangled hair, razor cuts, minor burns, twisted angles, hangnails, and most tension headaches have at least one factor in common—they are all examples of acute pain.

All of us have experienced acute pain in our lives, usually as the result of some routine daily activity that suddenly goes wrong. Acute pain serves as a warning that something somewhere in the body is amiss and requires immediate attention. Though a headache may last all day and a twisted ankle may hurt for a week, acute pain does have a time limit. The limit can be the instant that it takes to pull a comb through the knot in your hair or the time needed for a mashed finger to mend. The discomfort may be severe but we can take comfort in the knowledge that it will be alleviated in time.

Acute pain also serves a protective function. Accidentally placing your finger on a hot oven will produce an instantaneous "jerk reflex" as the hand is quickly removed. Your finger may blister and hurt, but there is really little to worry about. Acute pain, by definition, gets better.

Acute pain is also very closely associated with the psychological state of anxiety. Your burned finger produced not only pain, but a "full body alert," including a protective jerk reflex, generalized muscle tension, adrenalin released into the bloodstream, fear, and increases in both your heart rate and rate of respiration—symptoms considered to be in keeping with the state we generally term anxiety. Your mashed finger quickly pulled from the automobile undoubtedly produced a moment of fear, if not panic, and anxiety as you surveyed the bloody damage. Acute pain may result in anxiety but, like the pain, the psychological state of anxiety usually disappears as the discomfort is reduced.

When pain lasts for six months or longer of periodic or unremitting episodes, it can be decisively defined as chronic in nature. Chronic pain does not serve as a warning for the body to take action. In fact, unlike acute pain, chronic pain serves no useful purpose. Whereas acute pain can usually be tied to a source, the causes of chronic pain are often uncertain. Whereas acute pain is a symptom of an identifiable disorder, chronic pain is more correctly described as a disease in itself, rather than as a symptom of something else. Unlike acute pain, chronic pain may never fully cease. In fact, it often gets worse. Chronic pain can be continuous, 24 hours a day, seven days a week, 365 days a year. The intensity of pain may vary, but one factor remains constant: the pain is always present.

While acute pain is generally associated with anxiety, chronic pain is usually accompanied by depression. Research has indicated that depression and chronic pain may be related in two important ways. First, a depressed individual is statistically more prone to suffer a painful injury and, once in pain, the depression seems to prolong the suffering. Certainly it is true that individuals hospitalized in psychiatric facilities for depression also report pain complaints in numbers that far exceed statistical probability. Many individuals who suffer chronic pain do not recognize the severity of their depression and mislabel their problem as pain when, in fact, the primary disorder is intense depression. I occasionally see patients in my practice who have received numerous diagnostic evaluations and treatments for chronic pain and who deny any significant level of depression. Yet when psychotherapy and medication for depression are instituted, they experience marked pain relief. Not everyone suffering chronic back pain is suffering a primary depression, but significant emotional distress can occasionally herald the onset of pain.

Depression may also exist as a logical result of suffering chronic pain. This type of depression is termed *reactive depression* and becomes a factor as the pain sufferer gradually experiences an emotional "wear and tear" as the result of intractable pain. Reactive depression can also complicate effective management of chronic pain and should be recognized and appropriately dealt with by both the pain victim and health-care practitioner.

PHYSIOLOGICAL MECHANISMS OF PAIN

Physiology of Pain

The perception we commonly refer to as pain involves the entire central nervous system: the brain, spinal cord, and miles of nerves in the body. The central nervous system controls the *voluntary* muscles, such as those used in walking, riding a bicycle, driving a car, and playing tennis. However, the experience of pain also involves the sympathetic nervous system, a part of the autonomic nervous system. The autonomic nervous system controls the "automatic," or *involuntary*, muscles of the body, such as the heart muscle and the muscles that assist in breathing. The sympathetic nerves travel to all the arteries in the body, which, in turn, control the amount of blood flow to the muscles.

Nerves serve an important function in the body since they act as pain receptors, picking up pain messages much like a radio antenna picks up radio waves. Pain begins as a stimulus that is then picked up by the nerves. Once a pain stimulus or message is received by the nerve ending, it is carried to the brain and back again to the affected body part by the nerves.

Nerves are made up of tiny nerve cells that receive and forward pain messages. Each cell has a receiver end called a dendrite and a transmitter end called an axon. Pain messages travel as an electrical impulse from the axons of one cell to the dendrites of the next, and so on down the line. The gap between the axons and dendrites is called a synapse, and it is here that pain messages are deciphered and coded. Depending on the type of chemical coating, a pain message reaching a synapse may be terminated completely, changed and rerouted in some way, or simply forwarded to the neighboring cell.

This "decision" at the synapse is influenced strongly by chemical substances called neurotransmitters that are activated by pain messages. Neurotransmitters also assist in the pain-message transmission since they "bridge the gap" between axons and dendrites. A number of different neurotransmitters have been identified, including serotonin, dopamine, norepinephrine, and acetylocholine. This transmission process, however, can be reduced or increased by drugs. In fact, many medications are designed purposely to alter the transmission of electrical impulses across the synapse and can therefore serve as an aid in pain control. We will learn more of this in Chapter 7.

Many researchers believe that pain messages travel from the body to the brain on one of two "superhighways." The pain message starts with a stimulus and travels up the spinal cord; this is called the spinothalamic tract. Once the message gets to the brain, it meets a fork in the road. One highway travels through portions of the brain called the thalamus and hypothalamus to the limbic system. Called the paleospinothalamic tract, this is the tract on which pain that has been described as a steady ache or dull ache travels. The other highway is called the neospinothalamic tract. Sharp, stabbing impulses usually travel this highway to the brain.

Biochemistry of Pain

Another important part of the overall experience of pain is the influence of biological chemicals in our body and how these chemicals serve either to increase or decrease the level of pain that we feel. This has been a topic of much interest and debate in scientific circles over the past several years. Unfortunately, while there exists a great deal of speculation, there is little fact.

In the past few years, most investigative efforts into the biochemical influence of pain have focused on the importance of protein substances called *neurokinins* and the role they play in reducing pain thresholds. Many researchers believe that the experience of pain triggers the release of neurokinins in the body, thus increasing the discomforting quality of pain. A simple way to think of the role of neurokinins is to imagine a dam and reservoir. Under most conditions neurokinins are safely stored in the body much like water backed up by a dam. However, under certain conditions, such as heavy and prolonged rain, the dam can break, causing flooding and greatly complicating a bad situation. When pain is experienced, not only is there the problem of discomfort, but the pain may somehow "break the dam" and release a flood of neurokinins, which in turn increase the pain.

One neurokinin theory postulates that the substances are released when tissue cells in the body are damaged or destroyed. The release of neurokinins then concentrates around nerve endings and fibers involved in the transmission of pain signals from a body part to the brain. As the pain signals travel up a nerve, neurokinins "amplify" the pain signal.

A similar process has been known to occur in migraine head-aches. In the early stage of migraine development, another bio-chemical, serotonin, is released in the body. Serotonin causes vasoconstriction (arteries in the head decrease their diameter and allow less blood flow). Constriction of the cephalic arteries (located in the head area) and decreased blood flow are thought by many researchers to cause the "flashing lights" and uneasy lightheaded feeling known as prodromals that many migraine victims suffer prior to the onset of severe pain. Once the serotonin is depleted, however, the arteries become more flexible, the body is flooded with a release of neurokinins, and the arteries dilate in throbbing, excruciating pain. The presence of neurokinins is thought to lower the threshold at which the throbbing arterial dilations are felt as painful.

Endorphins

Not only does it seem very likely that the body manufactures biochemicals such as neurokinins that amplify the intensity of pain, but recent research has also identified pain-reducing biochemicals produced in the human body. These substances are called endor-phins, and many researchers believe they represent an important component in the body's own mechanism for controlling pain.

Endorphins have a number of similarities to potent narcotic pain-killing drugs such as morphine (Chapter 7). For example, endor-phins are nearly identical to morphine in chemical structure. In addition, endorphins, like morphine, exert their chemical action by blocking a number of important transmission sites in the central nervous system. This alteration in nerve transmission seems to de-crease the intensity and quality of pain. Finally, endorphins are thought to act on the same special cells in the brain and spinal cord that the opiate narcotic drugs attach to in order to produce an an-algesic and euphoric effect. Commonly known as opiate receptor cells, these cells seem to have a special affinity for man-made nar-cotic drugs. This affinity led researchers to suspect the existence of endorphins even before they were formally identified.

If you seem to have a lower threshold for pain than other people, perhaps your body has a deficiency of endorphins or receptor cells. Research in this area is continuing to document the important role of endorphins in the experience of pain. Endorphins may be pre-scribed some day to treat chronic back pain, depression, and other related disorders. To harness the human body's pain-reducing chemicals for use in treating medical disorders would solve a giant portion of the puzzle of pain.

Gate Control Theory

In 1965 Drs. Ronald Melzack and Patrick Wall proposed a theory to explain how pain messages travel up the spinal cord to the brain. While the accuracy of this theory remains a topic of debate, there is little doubt that their theory, known as the "gate control theory," represents the most important theoretical contribution to the field of pain research.

The gate theory suggests that a specialized group of nerve cells in the spinal cord act as a control mechanism similar to a valve or gate. The gate regulates the flow of pain messages into the central nervous system from peripheral nerves. When the gate is open, pain messages pass through to the brain and register pain. When the gate is closed, pain messages do not pass through and, theoretically, pain should not be experienced.

According to Drs. Melzack and Wall, small bundles of nerve fiber keep the gate open, and larger nerve-fiber bundles, whose messages travel faster than the messages on the smaller bundles, can close the gate. This may partially explain why a painful back, leg, hand, or other body part seems to hurt less when we rub the area. For example, if you pinch your finger in a desk drawer, the pain will slowly travel up small nerve-fiber bundles toward the brain. If you briskly rub your finger and hand, the response of rubbing will initiate a faster message along large nerve-fiber bundles, signaling the gate to close and limiting the amount of pain you experience.

We know that psychological variables also play an important role in regulating the flow of pain messages through the gate. We may closely attend to the pain or use distraction techniques to keep our minds off pain. In addition, the expectation and stress of pain have an impact on the function of the gate. The gate control theory represents an important pioneering theory to explain the experience of pain as a psychobiological phenomenon.

PSYCHOLOGICAL MECHANISMS OF PAIN

Tension, Stress, and Pain

Anatole France once said, "In all the world, the unhappiest creature is man." There are few times when we are completely happy. Throughout our lives worries persist—school, work, responsibilities, indebtedness, getting enough to eat, having shelter over our heads, war, success, and a host of other considerations.

The wards of any psychiatric hospital are full of people lying about with knees drawn up, backs tilted forward, and curled up as though they were in their mothers' wombs—safe, warm, and secure. Their unconscious minds want to escape back to that time when all was right, peaceful, and tranquil. They want to shut out the troublesome world by keeping their eyes closed and covering their heads.

There are times when the rest of us would also like to escape from the tensions, turmoil, and stress of everyday living. But we are simply unable to do so. As a result we often pay a heavy price in illness and symptoms.

Very few symptoms are significant if they occur only once in a while in a fleeting way, but when they return with unusual frequency, then the intelligent victim will beware. Here are some common signs of tension and stress that should be reviewed and remembered:

1. Habitually grinding one's teeth, tightening one's lips, or biting one's nail.

2. Being suspicious of people, mistrustful of friends, and carrying a chip on the shoulder.

3. Receiving little or no satisfaction from life's small joys.

4. Being chronically tired, with no great physical exertion to account for it, or finding it hard to get to sleep or stay asleep.

5. Becoming intensely angry over small irritations and minor disruptions in daily schedules.

When tension and stress become greater than we can tolerate, they take their toll on our bodies through a variety of psychologically induced symptoms and responses. The tension and stress are alleviated by being channeled through the nervous system to the organs of the body—which may then manifest in heart, stomach, or skin problems; respiratory ailments, such as asthma or hyperventilation; obesity; headaches; sexual difficulties; or, of course, back pain.

It is well known that stress, tension, and other psychological variables can serve as precipitating factors in serious back pain. Try this experiment: Make a tight fist and hold the muscle tension in your hand for a few minutes. After a minute or so, your hand will begin to hurt and a few minutes later you will experience rather severe pain.

The same principle holds true for the back. When we are stressed or experience prolonged tension and anxiety, the muscles throughout the body tense. Because the back is such a rich and large area of musculature, very severe back pain can frequently result. The pain mechanism in "tension headaches" is the same—muscles throughout the head, neck, and shoulders tense in response to stress and anxiety and ultimately cause pain. A recent experiment in Seattle, Wash., graphically demonstrated the important role of stress and tension in causing back pain. A woman whose back had been hurting for over five years, with numerous physicians unable to identify a significant cause for her problem, was hooked up to an EMG biofeedback unit with electrodes applied to her back muscles. As will be discussed in Chapter 10, EMG biofeedback measures the amount of muscle tension in a targeted muscle or muscle group. The investigator next conversed with the woman on numerous topics and noticed an interesting result. When the investigator brought the conversation around to the woman's domineering and querulous mother and to the husband, who, like the mother, was demanding and unsympathetic, the muscle tension in the back greatly increased. Within minutes the woman was complaining of increased back pain. When the conversation was later switched to some neutral topic, the muscles relaxed and the woman reported a decrease in her pain intensity. A total of 65 subjects with back pain were tested in this investigation and only one was found to have a totally organic or physical cause for back pain.

In addition to prolonged anxiety and tension as a cause of back pain, depression is also a psychological factor that frequently results in complaints of pain. The depressed individual is often totally unaware of suffering serious depression. While the individual knows that something is wrong because of back pain and a feeling of weakness and fatigued, he or she is usually the last to realize that the pain is the result of depression.

A man I treated during my internship training exemplified this pain pattern. A pleasant supervisor at a local factory, he was referred to me with a diagnosis of "back pain of seven months' duration with no identifiable physical cause." I carefully explained a program of relaxation exercise and enrolled him in physical therapy for stretching and conditioning exercises. I recall feeling confident that in three or four weeks his backache would be a thing of the past.

Two weeks later he returned to my office for follow-up and reported a decrease in his pain and claimed that the relaxation exercises and physical therapy seemed to be helping. But two weeks following he was back to see me with a report of increased pain and no relief from the treatment program. The next several months were characterized by inconsistent reports from my patient of improvement and no improvement, and I began to sense a growing irritation on my part. I had been taught how physical symptoms can sometimes mask a depression and became convinced that this was the cause of my patient's pain. Unfortunately, like most new doctors, I half believed that depressed individuals with complaints of pain were "really" aware of what they were doing and could pull themselves together once they knew I was onto their game. This patient taught me to appreciate the compelling role that the unconscious plays in our lives—a lesson I shall never forget.

Although long overdue, I sat down with my patient to talk. Within an hour I learned that he was excessively defensive about his pain. The longer he had pain with no identified physical diagnosis, the more suspect his problem had become. During the course of our conversation some revealing things came to light. I found out that all his life he had felt obligated to do more than his share. Because he did not think much of himself, he had to work harder than others to build up his self-esteem. Always running in high gear, he had little reserve physical or psychological strength. Shortly before he began having back pain, his wife had told him about a flirtation she had had with another man. This news further confirmed my patient's belief that he was worth little as a man. The patient became depressed, his job performance suffered, and before long he received a reprimand at work and sank into depression even further. It was at about this time that my patient began experiencing back pain.

This individual's pain started at a time when he was emotionally depleted. He had apparently transferred all his anger and disappointment with his wife and job into low back pain—a more socially acceptable complaint than depression. Furthermore, he was plagued with an unrealistic self-concept and pessimistic thoughts about the future.

The story had a happy ending. The patient gradually accepted the idea that his back pain was being caused by psychological depression. Over the next several office visits, he and his wife learned that his overworking made her feel neglected, while her flirtations–no matter how innocuous they really were–could do nothing but undermine the marriage and add to his depression and pain. The patient ultimately learned to control his depression and pain and I learned to appreciate more fully the role of psychological variables in pain.

Psychological Factors Aggravating Back Pain

Not only can emotional stress, tension, anxiety, and depression cause physical pain, but the reverse is true as well. Most people, I think, recognize that there is a close relationship between the mind and body, and that to attempt to separate the two completely would be a frustrating and impossible task. Pain is never just a physical problem, yet I have found that many people with back pain do not realize, or will not acknowledge, the extent to which their emotions can contribute to their pain. Just as emotions can cause physical illness, they can determine our reaction to illness, and this reaction plays a major role in the amount of pain we suffer.

Let us see how psychological factors can aggravate physical back pain. This can happen in at least four ways, which I term tension and stress, concentration and expectation, learning, and compensation.

Tension and Stress

Tension and stress are normal conditions; your body could not function without them. Infants are born under significant stress and the competing athlete often exerts maximum cardiovascular and muscular stress. Even the anticipation of a long-awaited vacation trip or "that first kiss" as a youngster creates tension and stress. Tension and stress can be positive or negative. It is not the conditions of tension and stress themselves that create problems for us, but the way in which we perceive the conditions that ultimately spells the difference between a positive and negative effect.

Consider, for example, two friends involved in an automobile accident on their way to town for a shopping trip. Both women suffer broken legs and both are confined to bed for four weeks. The first victim is miserable with her feelings of guilt over her inability to take care of her family and responsibilities and struggles with a distressing sense of urgency to hasten the recovery. She becomes anxious and depressed. She hates the pain she suffers and hates herself for being involved in the accident. In total, she reacts to her situation with negative tension and stress and is, in a word, *miserable!*

The second victim of the unfortunate accident adapts to the unavoidable situation much differently. She uses her enforced spare time to telephone old friends, catch up on reading, and learn to cross-stitch, a skill she had long wanted to develop but for which she had never had the time.

Which of these two accident victims do you suppose suffered the greatest amount of pain? If you choose the first woman, you are correct. The reason is simple—negative emotional tension and stress create in the body a state of prolonged muscular tension and generalized arousal that serves to increase the perception of pain. I have termed this phenomenon the "feedback loop of pain." As can be seen in Figure 3-1 page 44, pain can result in heightened physiologic and cognitive arousal, a state we can term tension. Tension, in turn, leads to increased muscular and mental distress, which leads to increased pain, which leads to even greater physiologic and cognitive arousal, and so on. Like a snowball rolling down a hill, the feedback loop of pain can result in a steadily increasing pain problem. In addition to the pain problem, the individual experiences a deeper and deeper sense of despair, tension, and misery—and intensified pain.

In later chapters, you will learn how to avoid the feedback loop of pain or, if already a victim, how to break the negative spiral of tension and stress that contributes to your pain.

Concentration and Expectation

A fact that few of us fully realize is the important role that selective concentration plays in our everyday lives. Routinely our minds screen out hundreds of impulses that constantly bombard our senses. This enables us to concentrate on whatever is important to us at the moment. If you are watching an interesting movie, your mind may focus your attention so that you are oblivious to the humming of the ventilation system, the whispering of the couple behind you, the hardness of the auditorium chair, or even the taste of the popcorn you unconsciously munch. If the movie is interesting enough, your attention may be so strong that almost nothing will disrupt your concentration.

Often, however, we are inclined to concentrate on pain, and sometimes it is to the exclusion of everything else. It is like running your tongue over a sensitive tooth even when you know the action will hurt. The more we concentrate on pain, the more pain we feel, and the more pain we feel, the more we expect to hurt.

It is well established that if you expect something to hurt, it probably will. Again, we emphasize the complex relationship between the mind and body. Consider, for example, this 1889 medical report from the physician Dr. C. Lloyd Tuckey:

There are few cases of this kind more remarkable than one related by Mr. Woodhouse Braine, the well-known chloroformist. Having to administer ether to an hysterical girl who was about to be operated on for the removal of two sabaceous tumors from the scalp, he found that the ether bottle was empty, and that the inhaling bag was free from even the odor of any anesthetic. While a fresh supply was being obtained, he thought to familiarize the patient with the process by putting the inhaling bag over her mouth and nose, and telling her to breathe quietly and deeply. After a few inspirations, she cried, "Oh, I feel it; I am going off," and a moment after, her eyes turned up, and she became unconscious. As she was found to be perfectly insensible and the ether had not yet come, Mr. Braine proposed that the surgeon should proceed with the operation. One tumor was removed without in the least disturbing her, and then, in order to test her condition, a bystander said that she was coming to. Upon this she began to show signs of waking, so the bag was once more applied, with the remark, "She'll soon be off again," when she immediately lost sensation and the operation was successfully and painlessly completed. (*Mastering Pain*, Feuerstein & Skjel, 1979, p. 34)

Further substantiating the powerful influence of expectation in our experience of pain is the phenomenon of placebo drugs. Placebos are usually plan salt or sugar pills with no active ingredients, yet the placebo effort on pain is often remarkable. Patients taking them are given the suggestion that the placebos are powerful and effective drugs. For many pain patients, the expectation of relief produces pain relief that approaches the effectiveness of the most powerful analgesic drugs.

The role of pain intensity and expectation can also have an opposite effect. In one study subjects were given a description of what was to occur. The first description did not include the word "pain" or "painful," whereas the second description did. As you might guess, the second shock was consistently rated as more painful than the first, even though the intensity of two was the same.

In cases of chronic back pain, it is the ongoing nature of the disease that alters our expectations. The depression and frustration of living in constant distress can soon deplete our optimism and expectations for relief. In time, we come to expect pain, and as our expectation of pain increases, so too does our pain.

It soon becomes a cycle–the more we hurt, the more we expect to hurt; the more we expect to hurt, the more we hurt; and so on. Breaking the cycle of pain and expectation requires a determined and consistent effort. Throughout this book you will find many helpful hints to help you modify your attitude toward pain in order to become the master of your back discomfort rather than the victim of your pain.

Learning

Physical pain is capable of generating a wide range of conscious and unconscious emotional responses, and one emotional response can often generate many others. This danger is, of course, not as great with the simple, short-lived attack of acute back pain as it is with chronic, long-lasting discomfort. A repeatedly documented and scientifically verified fact that at first may prove difficult fully to comprehend is this—human beings can "learn" to hurt. Now before closing your mind to this seemingly bizarre idea, consider two important facts of human behavior. The first is that each of us is inclined to continue any activity that is rewarded or reinforced in some manner. The second is that we are also inclined to continue any activity of behavior that allows us to avoid or escape an unpleasant situation. We go to work each day in part because we are rewarded with a paycheck. We smile and speak to individuals in passing, particularly physically attractive individuals, partly because we are usually rewarded with a returned smile and greeting. We seek to engage in sexual activity because we are most often rewarded with the pleasantness of the activity and orgasm. We pay our bills each month to avoid the unpleasantness of living without heat and electricity. We may be "forced" to work long and hard extra hours at the office on a "special" project on the weekend that our least favorite out-of-town relatives arrive for a weekend visit. We may be especially kind and thoughtful to old Uncle Jim because we hope eventually to be financially rewarded in his will. The laws of behavioral psychology clearly tell us that behaviors that are rewarded or reinforced by allowing us to get something we desire or avoid something we do not want are likely to increase in frequency, intensity, and duration.

But what has all of this to do with pain? Just as your mind and body react in the production of pain, so too can you and your family interact in ways to aggravate your condition. Your family may do you, and themselves, a disservice by showing too much, or too little, concern about your back pain.

Overconcern ironically, is a big danger for the person who is the ever-reliable, workaholic, anchorperson for a family. These individuals often work at two jobs to provide for the family and then volunteer for the local rescue squad. They spend years serving their family without letup—never sick, never taking a day off, always there to lend a helping hand, and serving as the indestructible "pillar of the family."

Cast in the role, anyone is likely to experience psychological difficulties with a prolonged pain problem. The attack may be entirely physical at the outset, but Mr. or Ms. Indestructible develops a new need: the need to express the fear of what is wrong. Yet this individual has never allowed himself or herself to show any weakness. The double bind is the inability either to talk about the agony and despair, or to dismiss it. The previously unsolicitous spouse and family rally around the victim, convinced that whatever is wrong must be terribly serious because nothing short of catastrophic pain could slow down this seemingly indestructable person. The family suddenly takes care of every need, fufilling the victim's every wish, feeding the person in bed or a favorite chair, changing the television channel, and huddling together around the victim eagerly awaiting the next desire to be expressed.

Through this newly demonstrated caring and attention are very pleasant, eventually, the victim is on the spot. Subconsciously, the victim recognizes that the family's new expectation must be lived up to if the devoted concern and pampering are to continue. The only way to do that is to continue suffering debilitating pain. Pain and suffering have been reinforced and rewarded.

Ironically, the same psychological response–subconsciously intensified pain–can occur if a family displays too little concern for a back pain victim's problem. A person who suffers pain naturally expects some assistance and attention. If the family seems indifferent, the victim may be too considerate or too proud to demand that attention. And so the body makes the demand instead, by producing a convincing degree of pain. The message is, "I really am in terrible agony. Now everyone has to notice me." Frequently these individuals will walk with a severely exaggerated limp or will insist on using a self-prescribed walking cane or crutches.

Finally, we know that we are likely to continue any behavior that allows us to avoid or escape an unpleasant situation. Consider the back pain victim who can manage, with the aid of a walking cane, friends, and a great deal of suffering and determination, to travel 30 miles to attend a football game or go fishing because "the doctor said I should try to get out and do a few things." However, this same individual "hurts too badly" to drive across town to see a less-than-favorite relative or to report to work on Monday morning.

It is important to keep in mind that the examples of learned pain as described should not be interpreted as the victim faking the pain. Malingering is not a question in cases of chronic learned back pain. You must remember that learned pain takes place *outside* your conscious control. Your back pain usually starts out as a physical problem, as the result of injury or repeated misuse. But in time your mind and back simply gang up on you to get what most of us want and need–more attention, more rest, more help, and more understanding. Unfortunately, you pay the price in continuing back pain.

As you have probably surmised by now, you can avoid the hazards of learned pain by understanding these psychological processes in advance. Once you are aware of them, you will see the value in expressing yourself directly and clearly, so that your body will not have to convey your message by intensifying pain. If you feel you may already be a victim of learned pain, do not despair! It does not mean that you are weird, susceptible, or crazy. You are simply the victim of a normal learning process, a process that every individual is subject to given the proper circumstances and situation. Throughout the remainder of this book will be found techniques for breaking the tight grip of learned pain.

Compensation

No chapter devoted in part to the psychological factors aggravating back pain would be complete without a section on the role that financial compensation plays in injury and pain. Sometimes, especially when money is involved, people in positions of authority may encourage you to maintain your dependence on pain and suffering. If you are involved in a lawsuit over a back injury, this may be done inadvertently, in the normal preparation of your case. Your lawyer will call you up from time to time and ask, "How's your back?" You may not have experienced a great deal of back pain in the past several weeks, but given the time, effort, and expense that have gone into the preparation of your case, you are not about to embarrass your lawyer or yourself by getting better too soon. The last thing you're inclined to say is, "Drop the case, my back is much better."

A lawyer may also unintentionally encourage you to prolong your pain as a cautionary measure: "We don't want to settle until you're completely pain-free." Such advice may be ethical and responsible legal practice but it does little to help you back to a more normal and productive life-style.

Compensation boards and worker's compensation insurance plans can be even more damaging in encouraging you to continue in pain. That is not what the system was intended to do or what the individuals who run the system intend to do, but it is simply an inherent flaw in the system. Instead of encouraging and motivating you to manage your pain and return to work, the system rewards you for hurting and disability and punishes you for feeling better.

If you are a victim of chronic pain and receive compensation for your suffering, it might pay you to examine your motives, privately and honestly, to make sure that "the system" and unintentional encouragement from others have not resulted in giving you a "need" for your pain. The compensation system is a morally just and humane system but it does have an undeniable potential for abuse. Lawyers are generally ethical and responsible individuals who attempt to assist their clients as best they can. Yet the practice and expertise of lawyers lie in protecting your legal rights, which is not always best for you from a medical and psychological point of view. Utilize the system properly and beware of the pitfalls!

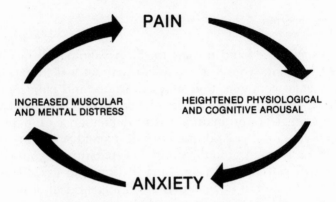

Figure 3-1—The two types of pain, acute and chronic, differ greatly in many aspects.

4

WHY BACKS HURT

Back pain is often a disorder of complex origins and symptoms. It is an indiscriminate enemy. It can originate in the muscles from some identified trauma, or have a nontraumatic onset. It can even begin elsewhere in the body and later attack the muscles. It can be neural in origin, emanating from the nerves and the nervous system. Back pain can also result from postural difficulties, congenital disorders, trauma, infections, degenerative disorders, inflammatory diseases, circulatory disorders, or from any of over 30 other different causes. And because of the profound complexity of the spine, the health professional investigating the cause of backache is often confounded by the inability of standard diagnostic tests and physical examination to pinpoint the exact cause of pain. The reason is simple—the human spine is a composition of bone, disk, muscle, ligament, tendon, and various other tissues organized in a labyrinth of portals, twists, turns, curves, and projections. This puzzling and intricate network can easily mask the cause of back pain in a perplexing arrangement and functioning of human physiology.

Complicating the identification of the cause of back pain even further is the unquestionable fact that there also exists an emotional component in human responses that can compound any physical disorder and intensify how much pain we perceive. The "psychology" of pain, introduced in Chapter 3, can mask the true cause of back pain. Depression, anxiety, frustration, reinforcement, stress, anger, fear, and a host of other psychological states can serve to: (1) herald the onset of back pain, (2) result as a normal reaction to a prolonged pain problem, or (3) exist concurrently with pain. In any case, the emotional component can greatly complicate the diagnosis of back pain, sometimes resulting in needless surgery and disability, while at other times masking the underlying physical causes of pain from even the most astute specialist. Look at the case of a young man named Al.

Al was a young man in his early 30s who had suffered emotional problems since he was a teenager. Despite several psychiatric hospitalizations and lengthy psychiatric treatment, he was unable to hold a steady job or lead a normal life. He would land a menial job and work for several months before a recurrent bout of severe agitated depression would render him disabled for months at a time. His ability to cope with life was marginal at best.

One day Al visited his family doctor complaining of low back pain. He gave the doctor a history of simply waking a week before with discomfort that had grown steadily more severe. Fully aware of Al's lengthy emotional problems, his doctor examined him, found no suggestion of organic problems, reassured him that the pain would go away, and sent him home.

Two weeks later Al returned to the doctor's office with complaints of steadily increasing back pain. His doctor again examined him and found nothing to explain the pain. The doctor sat down with Al, explained that his pain was part of his psychological problem, suggested he increase his dose of Valium to calm his anxiety, and sent him home.

Ten weeks later, with unrelenting pain, Al visited a local internist. The scenario was the same—four office visits over the next nine weeks, no objective findings to explain his pain physically, reaffirmed diagnosis of psychological pain, and reassurance that his pain would go away if only he would forget it and relax.

Al had now been in pain for over five months and was genuinely experiencing increased anxiety, depression, and frustration. He was unable to sleep and was rapidly losing weight. He was swallowing large quantities of Percodan tablets, supplied by a friend, in order to ease his pain and his psychological status deteriorated as his drug dependency strengthened and his pain persisted. It was now impossible to determine how much of Al's psychological problems existed prior to the onset of pain and how much depression and anxiety existed because of his back pain.

Taken to a psychiatrist's office by his concerned family, Al was immediately hospitalized in a local psychiatric hospital with a diagnosis of narcotic addiction and agitated depression. The next month passed slowly as Al was gradually withdrawn from Percodan. His complaints of back pain fell on deaf ears as treatment was targeted toward drug withdrawal and his emotional stability. The psychiatrist, tired of the persistent complaints, finally asked an orthopedic surgeon to examine Al. The diagnosis—"probable lumbar strain with strong psychological factor."

After a year of painful suffering, narcotic dependency, psychiatric hospitalization, and five different physicians, Al saw a orthopedic surgeon who suggested a brief hospitalization for diagnostic tests, including a myelogram, CAT scan, and psychological studies (Chapter 6). The myelogram was normal, but the CAT scan suggested a herniated lumbar disk. Psychological studies suggested that while Al did suffer significant problems with anxiety and depression, the likelihood of his pain being caused by his emotional problems was minimal. The decision was made to perform a surgical procedure known as diskectomy (Chapter 9).

Al experienced immediate postsurgical relief. Two months later he was back at work, his pain eliminated and his psychological state calm.

Al is typical of countless individuals whose back pain problems somehow fall through the crack of traditional medical diagnostic systems. While some individuals do develop various physical problems, including back pain, as a result of psychological variables such as stress, tension, depression, and anxiety, the great majority gradually become afflicted with emotional difficulties while seeking pain relief, often for years. It is its emotional or psychological component that complicates our perception of pain and clouds the physician's assessment of symptoms and complaints, particularly doctors not specifically trained in the profound complexity of pain.

In Al's case the cause of his pain was threefold. The herniated disk was the cause of his initial pain. This physical component then was compounded by his emotional or psychological response—his anxiety and depression from not getting relief, the frustration at not finding a doctor who believed his complaints, and the restrictions placed on his life. Finally, Al's psychological state exacerbated his physical problems and caused him to experience greater pain. The "pain–tension cycle" initiated by tissue damage that leads to emotional difficulties and to increased perception of pain is common in chronic back pain patients (Chapter 3).

Let us examine some of the sources and most common causes of back pain. Perhaps you will find information consistent with your pain and symptoms.

TRAUMA

Trauma is the most frequent cause of back pain. Each day thousands of people injure their backs because of injudicious lifting, a fall, or some type of accident. In fact, the *Journal of Occupational Health and Safety* reports that "on any given day, seven and one-half million workers are under treatment for back pain resulting from an industrial injury or accident." Traumatic injuries are so prevalent in our society because the majority of us are in embarrassingly poor physical condition. For example, most back pain that results from muscle strain could be avoided by proper weight control, the use of proper body mechanics, a regular program of physical activity consistent with age and physique, and daily exercises to keep trim and keep the muscles in the back and abdomen in proper tone. Yet the majority of patients seen for complaints of back pain are obese and poorly conditioned.

In my own practice I seldom see a healthy young person or athlete with back pain. The primary reason is that these individuals are generally in excellent physical shape. However, after age 30 or so, most of us become less active physically and exercise only sporadically, if at all, and gain weight. This type of physical deterioration is an invitation to the onset of traumatic back pain.

Low back pain is also common in women who have had several pregnancies with excessive weight gain and who fail to recondition themselves with a proper exercise program after delivery. Poor muscle tone, obesity, and physical deterioration frequently serve as precursors to traumatic back pain.

Muscle Strain

Muscular pain probably accounts for more health complaints than any other single source of back pain. Because of the anatomy and structure of the body, the muscles in the lower back are particularly susceptible to severe strain or tearing, particularly in individuals with weakened muscles resulting from a sedentary lifestyle.

When the back muscles are torn or strained beyond their capability, there is thought to be very small microscopic bleeding into the muscle. This results in painful muscle spasm as the traumatized muscles contract and harden. To compound the problem, movement or activity causes pain that results in "guarding" (an involuntary protective reflex that produces muscle spasms in areas adjoining the injured muscles). Muscles that are tensed for prolonged periods, as in muscle spasm, can themselves cause pain, as is evidenced by "tension headaches" or making a tight fist and holding the muscle tension for several minutes. Restricted movement and resting the injured back often result in muscle and joint stiffness, which makes the disability even more difficult to tolerate. It is not uncommon to suffer a painful traumatic back strain and take to one's bed, only to wake the next morning to find that the muscles have stiffened and spasmed to the point where the intensity of pain is greatly increased and that to climb from the bed is an almost impossible task!

Tension, anxiety, and stress, all of which can generate muscle spasms, are other factors that can increase the discomfort of muscle strain. While spasms of the back muscles usually start with strain or trauma to the back, worrying about the injury, pain, or any of life's other stresses that accumulate in our daily lives can create tension spasms that further increase the perception of pain.

Though back strain and muscle spasms are relatively common, it is sometimes hard for doctors to find evidence that muscle strain and spasm is causing the problem; the spasm may not be present at the time of your medical examination and muscle strain cannot be seen on x-ray or other sophisticated medical diagnostic procedure. In fact, there exists no single conventional diagnostic procedure to determine back strain. The diagnosis of back strain is generally made following a thorough physical examination to rule out other possible causes of pain and a complete medical history (Chapter 5). If the doctor questions you about your life, answer as honestly as possible. Keep in mind that you may think that everything is great and not consciously realize you are under stress or tension, which can contribute to your pain.

Most back strains can be effectively managed with a program that combines rest, physical therapy, stretching exercises, and medication. Instruction in the proper use of the body, particularly the proper posture and technique for lifting, pushing, standing, and sleep, may also prove helpful in returning you to a more normal life-style.

Ligament Strain

The back, like other parts of the human musculoskeletal system, is rich with supporting tissue called ligaments. Ligaments attach muscles to bones and may be strained by such traumas as improper lifting or a sudden fall, and if the trauma is severe, ligaments may be torn. Since ligaments work with muscles to provide strength and support of the back and spine, a ligament tear can be a painful and agonizing injury.

Of particular value in the diagnosis of ligament strain is that very seldom is a normal ligament tender if it is palpated (pressed or touched with the fingers). Therefore, if a ligament is palpated by your doctor and you feel a sharp sudden pain, the chances are good that you have suffered ligament injury or, in some cases, damage to the bony back joint. Symptoms of persistent back pain caused by ligament strain are generally relieved by rest, although complete healing is often frustratingly slow.

Spondylolysis and Spondylolisthesis

Many authorities consider spondylolysis and spondylolisthesis to be traumatic stress fractures of a portion of spinal anatomy located on both sides of a vertebra. The vertebrae in the lower back are the most commonly affected. *Spondylolysis* can affect either one or both sides of the vertebra, although the fracture is not sufficient to allow any slippage of the vertebra. *Spondylolisthesis* is a bilateral defect in which a portion of the affected vertebra can actually "slip" forward, with the remaining vertebra generally remaining in the normal position.

Perhaps spondylolysis and sponlylolisthesis can be more easily understood if we consider a column of bricks neatly stacked, one on the other, with masonry concrete holding the bricks firmly in place. If the concrete cracks around one brick but the brick remains firmly in place and cannot be moved, we would have a situation roughly similar to spondylolysis. However, if the concrete cracks sufficiently so that the brick can actually slip back and forth while the other bricks remain in place, we would have a rough analogy to spondylolisthesis. From this can be seen why spondylolisthesis is occasionally referred to as "loose back."

While both spondylolysis and spondylolisthesis can be congenital, most authorities believe that in most cases they are traumatically acquired. However, there does seem to be a genetic factor involved. After the human body has reached sufficient anatomical maturity, generally after age five, or more commonly in teenage years, repeated shearing stresses such as occur in gymnastics or contact sports can cause a stress fracture in a part of the vertebra when there is a genetic predisposition. The fracture may then develop into one of these two defects. Of course, a fall or other trauma suffered at a later age can also potentially cause sufficient damage to result in either injury.

X-rays are generally sufficient to demonstrate the stress fracture of spondylolysis or the fracture and vertebral slippage of spondylolisthesis. While both disorders can cause back pain, spondylolisthesis more commonly results in the symptom of low back discomfort.

If your doctor diagnoses spondylolysis or spondylolisthesis, your treatment is likely to be conservative—rest, moderate exercise, instruction in body mechanics, mild analgesics, and physical therapy. In cases of spondylolisthesis, your physician may recommend periodic repeated x-rays if there is cause to suspect that the vertebral slippage may increase. Should the slippage continue and symptoms become increasingly intense, an operation termed spinal fusion (Chapter 9) may be necessary to prevent further slippage that could cause pressure on and stretching of the lumbar nerve roots with resulting neurologic problems, such as difficulty in walking and possible bowel or bladder problems. Such neurological problems are possible, but are generally quite rare.

Compression Fracture

Compression fractures usually result from a fall and, as a general rule, often affect the lower thoracic and upper lumbar vertebrae. X-rays of the spine will normally identify the fracture by the wedge-shaped appearance of the vertebra. Although the great majority of compression fractures of the spine respond well to bed rest, physical therapy, and conservative medical care, there does exist an outside possibility that secondary medical problems may occur. If you have symptoms suggesting the possibility of a compression fracture, a thorough neurological examination is necessary. Since underlying malignancy and osteoporosis (softening of bone) may make one more susceptible to compression fracture, these two disorders will be thoroughly investigated during your doctor's examination. In patients with osteoporosis, the trauma required to fracture a vertebra is often surprisingly trivial—sudden lifting of even a light object, a minor slip or fall, or, with one particular patient recalled, improper bending to tie a shoe.

DEGENERATIVE DISEASE

For our purposes back pain from degenerative diseases can be considered a "wear-and-tear" phenomenon. An analogy can be made to the deterioration of an automobile. The more a car is abused and the greater the stresses and strains imposed on it, the more it will squeak, rust, and rattle as it ages. Similarly, the human spine begins to "squeak and rattle" with increasing trauma, obesity, and age, sometimes causing back pain or setting the stage for other conditions that may give rise to back discomfort.

We will consider three relatively common disorders as degenerative in nature—osteoarthritis, spondylosis, and herniated or "slipped" or "ruptured" disk. Alone or, more often, in combination, they can lead to spinal stenosis and nerve root entrapment.

Osteoarthritis

An estimated 16 million people in the United States have osteoarthritis serious enough to cause pain. Perhaps as many as 30 million more would show evidence of the disease on an x-ray, but would not have significant symptoms. The occurrence of osteoarthritis increases with advancing age. When all ages are considered, women are affected about twice as frequently as men. If we live long enough, it is a safe bet that each of us will develop osteoarthritis to some degree.

Osteoarthritis has numerous names—degenerative joint disease, arthrosis, and osteoarthrosis—and is a disease of the joints that involves a breakdown of cartilage and other tissues that make a movable joint function properly. Osteoarthritis may affect practically any joint in the body, including the back, and the damage is inflamation, but pain and decreased normal motion sometimes occur. Do not confuse osteoarthritis with rheumatoid arthritis—rheumatoid arthritis causes inflamation of the joints and can affect the entire body, including the internal organs, while osteoarthritis does not affect the entire body and seldom causes inflamation.

The pain of spinal osteoarthritis is caused by irritation and pressure on nerve endings, muscle tension, and muscle fatigue. It is interesting to note that osteoarthritis pain is not always related to the amount of tissue damage present in a joint. For instance, an individual with a joint severely affected by osteoarthritis may experience less pain than other individuals with a joint that appears only mildly affected.

If you suspect that you may have osteoarthritic back pain, consult your physician. In most instances a careful analysis of symptoms and thorough examination of your back can give the doctor a good idea of the problem. When there is significant joint involvement, special tests may be necessary, both to confirm the diagnosis and to determine how serious the problem is. Often these tests are useful in ruling out other types of arthritis.

The most valuable diagnostic test for osteoarthritis probably is x-ray, which generally show characteristic changes associated with osteoarthritis. Another test, called sedimentation rate, measures how quickly red blood cells settle to the bottom of a small tube. The red blood cells from a person with chronic inflamation settle more rapidly than normal. Osteoarthritis patients without complicating illnesses have normal sedimentation rates. Sometimes blood counts are performed as part of an initial diagnostic examination, and at intervals when certain treatments are being administered.

It is important to know that while osteoarthritis cannot be cured, its symptoms can be alleviated and impaired joint function improved. Osteoarthritis is one of an increasing important number of chronic disorders for which treatment generally involves doing a number of things instead of just one or two, and is targeted toward management as opposed to cure. In general, the treatment for osteoarthritis consists of controlling pain and discomfort (either by drugs or other techniques described in this book) and protecting the joints from stresses and strain. Impaired joint function is treated by protecting the joint from stress by rest; by back braces and corsets;

by specific exercises to strengthen muscles, correct posture defects, and prevent misuse of a joint; and, in very rare and severe cases, by surgical operations.

Spondylosis

Spondylosis is a degenerative process that affects a spinal disk and that also creates changes in the vertebrae located above and below the affected disk. It is the most common disorder seen on x-ray in middle-aged and older individuals with low back pain. Frequently, spondylosis produces no pain or symptoms and is discovered by chance on spinal x-rays taken for other reasons. Many authorities believe that back pain caused by spondylosis is precipitated only when fatigue or injury interferes with the normal homeostatis status of the spine. Because spondylosis is so common and so frequently produces no symptoms, your doctor will generally not consider the disorder as the cause of your back pain until other possible causes are excluded.

If spondylosis is considered to be the cause of back discomfort, treatment is generally conservative—physical therapy, mild analgesics, and instruction in body mechanics and spinal care.

"Slipped" Disk and Sciatica

"Slipped," or "ruptured," or herniated disks, although relatively uncommon, are notorious for causing severe pain and disability. The various terms are used because the jellylike semisolid center of a disk (nuceleus pulposus) may "slip," shift, or bulge, or, in more advanced cases, may actually rupture (herniate) the disk encasement like a tire blowout. While individuals with this disorder usually claim pain from a traumatic injury such as in an industrial or automobile accident, most authorities believe the injury represents the "straw that broke the camel's back." In other words, the disorder is a degenerative long-term wear-and-tear process that finally culminates with traumatic injury and the onset of pain and symptoms. The fourth and fifth lumbar disks are most frequently affected.
confined to the joints and surrounding tissue. There is little or no

Disk herniation may exert direct pressure on a spinal nerve root and compress it, causing nerve irritation with pain along the parts of the body supplied by the affected nerve. In many cases of low back disk herniation, one or both of the legs also hurt. This can result in atrophy (wasting away of muscle tissue due to the interruption in nerve supply) and weakness in the muscles supplied by the affected nerve. Examination of any neurologic changes is part of a thorough medical examination (Chapter 5).

Individuals who suffer a herniated disk most commonly report severe low back pain developing immediately or a few hours after an injury. Often the victim, who is usually between the ages of 30 and 50, reports heavy lifting, a severe fall, or twisting motion while moving a heavy object. The pain, intensified by sneezing, straining, or forward bending, is associated with severe back muscle spasm.

Since the herniated disk can compress or pinch ("pinched nerve") one or more spinal nerve roots, the sufferer can also have *sciatica*. Sciatica is a name for pain that radiates along the course of the sciatic nerve—down the buttocks and back of the leg, thigh, and calf, and, many times, even into the foot. Paresthesia (tingling and prickling sensation) and numbness occur in over half the cases of herniated disk.

A disk herniation at a particular level of the spinal column produces a distinctive clinical picture because of the specific spinal nerve root involved. As a result a thorough physical examination usually indicates or gives strong suggestion of the involved disk. In fact, most classic cases of disk herniation can be diagnosed on the basis of the clinical history and physical examination alone. Specialized tests such as myelogram, CT scans, and electromyography (Chapter 5) are generally part of a thorough examination if the physical examination suggests a herniated disk.

Treatment of disk herniation depends on numerous factors, including how much herniated disk material has actually entered the spinal canal, how many spinal nerve roots have been compressed, neurologic abnormalities, and the disability and severity of pain. Many individuals with disk disorders respond well to the nonsurgical treatments presented in this text. A small percentage do require surgery or a new treatment technique termed chemonucleolysis (Chapter 9).

Spinal Stenosis

Degenerative diseases, such as spondylosis and osteoarthritis, may result in a condition known as spinal stenosis, or nerve root entrapment syndrome. Herniated disks, in which the jellylike center of the disk "slips" into the spinal canal and traps a spinal nerve root, are also considered to be a form of spinal stenosis. Spinal stenosis is the formation of bony growth called *osteophytes*, and subsequent narrowing of the central spinal canal or lateral canals (where spinal nerve roots exit), and this narrowing of the exit canal may cause pressure on the spinal nerves or "trap" the nerves and cause pain and other symptoms. Spinal stenosis most frequently affects the lower part of the back.

Stenosis of the central spinal canal characteristically produces somewhat vague and unusual symptoms. A common complaint is leg pain that intensifies with walking and is relieved with rest. Stenosis of the lateral canal, in contrast, most often results in only buttock and thigh pain, with no significant discomfort down the length of the leg. Either a myelogram or CAT scan will generally confirm the diagnosis of central spinal stenosis, while lateral spinal stenosis is usually diagnosed best with a CAT scan. Depending on the severity of pain and symptoms, the age and health of the victim, and a host of other variables, the pain and symptoms of spinal stenosis may be well managed with relaxation techniques, TENS, and cognitive pain management techniques described throughout this text. However, a small percentage of patients may require surgery to "bore out" or open the narrowed canal and free the trapped nerve root. As with all back disorders, every effort should be made to manage the pain and symptoms without surgery, unless an operation is absolutely necessary.

MECHANICAL PROBLEMS

Ever since human beings had the nerve to assume the upright position and become the "backbone" of society, their backs have suffered. Humans do not have the advantage of walking on all-fours, and so their lower backs must bear the brunt of the body's weight. When aging, obesity, poor posture, lack of exercise, stress, and loss of muscle tone are added, an already overly burdened back can begin to ache!

Posture

Correct posture is essential for a healthy back. Because of the strategic location and function of the back, when posture is incorrect and increased stress and weight all added to ill-prepared body parts, the back is usually first to send out the message of pain.

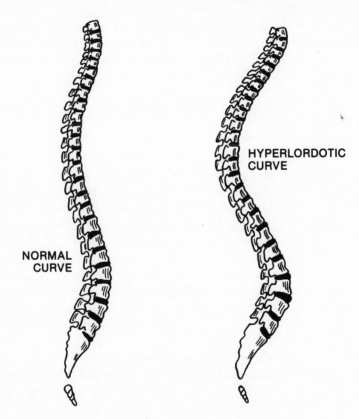

Figure 4-1—Normal and hyperlordotic spinal curves.

Hyperlordosis, a prime example, is a mechanical exaggeration of the normal curve in the lower back (Figure 4-1). With age, many people gain weight and lose muscle tone in the abdomen. As a result the abdomen and buttocks protrude. This postural shift crowds the verebrae and narrows the canal through which spinal nerve roots are located. This narrowing subsequently causes "pinching" of the nerve root at its point of exit, which in turn causes nerve root entrapment and spinal stenosis. The "pinched" nerve is relieved when the patient bends forward, separating the vertebrae and enlarging the nerve root canal. Typically, patients with hyperlordotic back pain report severe radiating pain through the buttocks and down the leg while in a standing position and relief from discomfort when sitting down or bending forward.

The treatment for hyperlordotic back pain is straightforward and simple—loss of weight, abdominal strengthening exercises, and instruction in correct posture. With a combination of these treatments, the pain of hyperlordosis can usually be effectively managed.

Lumbar Scoliosis

Lumbar scoliosis (lateral curve of the lumbar spine) in normal, healthy adults is not unusual, and frequently produces no pain or symptoms when the curve is minor. However, if scoliosis is not detected in adolescence, the condition can deteriorate and cause severe back pain and disability when the victim reaches adulthood. Originally it was thought that progressive scoliosis would halt when the patient reached skeletal maturity. However, it is now known that spinal curves in many adults progress one to two degrees each year, and perhaps five to eight degrees with each pregnancy. This progression may continue throughout adult life. Thus a victim with a ten-degree curve at age 18 may have a 40-degree curve and severe back pain before the age of 40.

Lumbar scoliosis is usually to the left side and is associated with an imbalanced pelvis. When the victim attempts to align the pelvis to correct the obliquity, the spine is tilted out of balance and the head no longer is centered over the pelvis. Over a period of time, this imbalance leads to degenerative spinal arthritis and low back pain.

Treatment for lumbar scoliosis ideally begins in adolescence and usually involves bracing the developing spine with corsets, braces, or casts to allow continued growth to correct the faulty curvature. In fact, in many cities local physicians and chiropractors perform free scoliosis and spinal examinations in the schools to detect spinal curvature in children, who usually respond well to treatment. When scoliosis is diagnosed after skeletal maturity, treatment is generally targeted toward postural training and pain control. Surgery may be required in a very small percentage of adults suffering progressive scoliosis and disability.

Fibromyalgia

Fibromyalgia (sometimes termed fibrositis) is a poorly understood rheumatic condition characterized by patient complaints of generalized muscle and joint aches and pains, chronic fatigue, and stiffness, predominantly in the lower back, shoulders, and knees. Other associated complaints include anxiety, sleep problems, headaches, irritable colon, subjective sense of swelling in the joints, and numbness. Often the condition is misdiagnosed as rheumatoid arthritis, psychogenic pain, neuritis, hypothyroidism, multiple sclerosis, and "nerves." Patients with this condition frequently suffer for years before an accurate diagnosis is made and appropriate treatment instituted.

The reason for misdiagnosis and mismanagement is that fibromyalgia is generally not recognized by physicians. In fact, there remains a small controversy over whether the condition even exists as a disease entity! This controversy and nonacceptance are caused by the fact that, until recently, there existed no standard criteria for diagnosis. As a result, fibromyalgia was not a diagnosis based on clinical evidence, but one that occasionally was offered when symptoms did not fit the criteria for any alternative diagnosis.

Fibromyalgia is most likely to affect women, and the majority are under 35 years of age at the onset of the problem. In most patients pain and stiffness vary during the day, becoming worse in the morning or evening, or both. Most victims report that the severity of pain varies with the weather and the degree of physical activity, fatigue, and anxiety. Laboratory tests are generally normal and the typical sufferer has gone from doctor to doctor and been told that there is nothing wrong. After a time, the victim begins to wonder if the pain and symptoms are all in the mind, and becomes depressed, which complicates the problem. Often its victims are subjected to potentially dangerous diagnostic techniques such as myelograms, arthrograms, and tests for cancer.

Recent medical studies suggest that fibromyalgia is becoming more clearly understood. There is now a general consensus that the diagnosis of fibromyalgia must be based on the composite picture, including the positive findings, and not simply rendered in the absence of other diseases. A key diagnostic feature is the presence of specific trigger points (localized areas of exaggerated tenderness to touch). The trigger points are most frequently located in the shoulder area and along the spine. When your doctor palpates (presses or touches) these trigger points, you will feel a sharp, intensified pain.

Treatment of fibromyalgia, similar to the treatment of most chronic pain conditions, is a team effort. Physical therapy modalities such as TENS, hot packs, and ultrasound may provide temporary relief in pain intensity. A regular program of physical exercise, including walking, stretching, and relaxation, also produces favorable results. If identified trigger points cause disabling pain, mild analgesic medication is used and the trigger points may be injected with a local analgesic. For the motivated and cooperative patient, the management of fibromyalgia pain is generally successful.

STRESS AND EMOTIONAL FACTORS

There is virtually no escaping it. If you are involved in life, you will encounter stress. Deadlines must be met and bills must be paid. You must face job pressures and fight traffic jams. Birthdays come and go. All of these events force you to adapt, to cope. All cause stress.

Unfortunately, though you may be able to put stressful events behind you one at a time, they have a way of accumulating and wearing on you over the years. After years of changing and adapting, your body and mind may be affected by the constant pressures. You may become chronically anxious and overstressed.

When you are put under pressure by a new or challenging situation, your body, in an effort to cope, responds by mobilizing forces to deal with this pressure. Chemicals pour into the bloodstream, your muscles tense, your heart rate increases, the blood flow to your brain increases, and you pull in greater quantities of oxygen. This is called the "fight-or-flight" response.

Thousands of years ago, when the challenges of life were real and tangible (an attack from the next village or from a wild animal), this reaction to stress was vital to survival. If your body responded fast enough, you were saved.

In modern society we still face stressful situations—some say more and stronger stresses than ever. Yet the *stressors*, as these events are called, are rarely as real as wild animals. Seldom do we get a chance to do direct battle with them. The damage comes if we do not learn to cope with the stressors. Inadequate coping can cause damage to our minds and bodies. Yet stress is inevitable in daily life, necessary, and often a positive force. The damaging effects of prolonged stress come not from the stressors, but our inability effectively to cope with the stressors.

The negative effects of stress can be numerous. Stress leads to anxiety, irritability, insomnia, and depression. It is a cause of headaches, backaches, and asthmatic attacks. In some people stress leads to heart disease, ulcers, high blood pressure, and many other serious health problems. Some recent studies have suggested a strong link between stress and certain cancers. To be sure, stress and anxiety can lead to increased muscular tension and pain.

The Emotional Back

It is difficult to generalize about human behavior, but we do know that certain general personality characteristics seem to be linked to greater pain tolerance, including effective stress-coping skills and lack of anxiety. On the other hand, two psychological states—depression and anxiety—go hand in hand with pain, and particularly chronic pain. Some pain researchers estimate that as many as half of all patients with chronic noncancerous pain are also significantly depressed and anxious. And not only does chronic pain tend to cause greater depression and anxiety, there is also the opposite tendency for chronically depressed and anxious individuals to be more vulnerable to painful disorders. In fact, it is frequently difficult to determine whether psychological disturbances in a person with pain are the *cause* of pain, the *result* of it, or are simply *concurrent* phenomena that have no causal relationship to pain at all, but are made more evident by the pain disorder and the attention it attracts. This is an example of the intricate psychological nature of pain.

If you feel that stress, anxiety, and other psychological variables may be a causal factor in your back discomfort *do not over react!* You are not an emotional cripple, a weak individual, or a psychiatric candidate, and, most important, the pain is *not* "all in your head." You are simply a victim of our pressure-packed contemporary society and the inhabitant of an evolutionary body designed to do life or death battle with wild animals, but living in a time when life or death threats are few. Consult your physician for a thorough physical examination, and then discuss the techniques for stress reduction, pain control, and physical conditioning described in this book. Pain *can* be successfully managed.

5

YOUR DOCTOR'S EXAMINATION

There's something unnerving about a doctor's office. It is a strange and anxiety-provoking place where a foreign language called "medical" is spoken. Visitors to this place sit patiently, waiting their turns to follow a nurse down a hall into a small windowless cubicle. Inhabitants (doctors and nurses) scurry up and down the halls, entering and quickly departing from similar cubicles. On looking around the small room, one is struck by the uncomfortable sterility of the environment, the confusing array of complex equipment, and the locked cabinets filled with strange "spirits," needles, and medications. Your back aches and you are a bit frightened. You feel out of your environment and out of control of your body and the situation. In time "Dr. Rushed," the self-proclaimed leader of this alien place, enters and begins asking questions about your back. At some point during the questioning, the doctor may stop writing and reading your chart and actually look you in the eye, usually for the first time since entering the room and usually some ten minutes into the questioning. Some of the questions do not seem to make sense and you wonder about the inquiry. The leader may next touch, pull, push, tug, lift, mash, tilt, twist, pinch, hit, jerk, tickle, and stretch your back and various other parts of your anatomy. Some of the maneuvers hurt. In fact, the doctor may repeatedly ask you throughout this tortuous ritual if different maneuvers hurt. It seems the doctor won't be satisfied until some motion is discovered that is guaranteed to bring tears to your eyes. This is all very confusing! Eventually satisfied that you have endured enough, the leader "explains" the suspected cause of your back pain. Unfortunately for those victims who don't speak "medical," the explanation is more confusing than enlightening. What is understood and remembered is the doctor's recommendation of "a few tests" and something about "pictures" and "needles." With the leader departed down the hall to deliver more healing wisdom, you are left alone in the cubicle with your confused thoughts. What was the doctor looking for? Why were all those questions asked? What are the diagnostic tests I should have? How are they performed? What was the doctor really saying was wrong with my back? Why did I endure this? What happens now?

If this sounds familiar, you are not alone. Each day thousands hobble into doctors' offices with aching, throbbing backs. Unfortunately many leave knowing little more than they did when the appointment was initially scheduled. If this has ever happened to you, there is no need for it ever to happen again. Let us spend a few minutes learning what your doctor looks for when you report back pain.

HISTORY

While the possible causes of back pain are many, the probable ones are relatively few. The chances are excellent that your doctor, with your help, can establish without much difficulty the reason for your discomfort. To pinpoint the cause of your pain, and to help rule out one cause from another (termed differential diagnosis), the doctor starts the investigation of pain with a thorough history.

The history will include a battery of questions that touch upon virtually every facet of your life. You will first be asked when the pain started, how it began, how severe it was, where it was located, whether the pain spread and where it spread to, and how the symptoms have changed since the onset. The doctor will want to know what makes the pain worse, what eases it, how frequently and for how long it hurts, if there are sensations of pins and needles or numbness, if weakness or stiffness has developed and when, whether coughing, sneezing, straining, or bowel movements increase the pain, and if the discomfort is relieved by rest. The type of work you do, and how satisfied you are with your job, your marriage, and home situation, are also factors that will be considered. The doctor will ask about anxiousness, depression, and stress, as well as your association with alcohol, cigarettes, drug consumption, and medications and their negative side effects. In addition, the doctor will be interested in your general health, what disease and medical problems you have had in the past, and if you are currently being treated for an active medical problem not associated with your back disorder. The questions may seem endless, but each bit of information assists the doctor in solving the puzzle of back pain.

Let us consider briefly the possible significance of only a portion of the information that can come from a thorough medical history. First, the severity of pain is not necessarily related to the seriousness of the cause. Many relatively minor back problems can cause pain that is as severe as that caused by more serious problems. However, certain types of irritative pain, such as that accompanying fracture of the spine or of a rib, are excruciating. Muscle spasm alone may be quite intense, but rarely to the point of being intolerable. A burning type of pain may indicate irritation of nerve fibers, while pins-and-needles (paresthesia) sensations may be due to interference with the blood supply, irritation of nerve roots by a tumor, or muscles and spasm. Back strain usually occurs with excessive physical stress on ligaments and muscles, is usually characterized by pain confined to the lower (lumbar) back, and is aggravated by movement. The sudden onset of low back pain following lifting, pushing, or pulling, followed in several days by a spreading, radiating pain in the leg, is often the result of a herniated disk. Gradually increasing low back pain with subtle radiation of discomfort into the leg, hip, or buttock may suggest degenerative disk disease. Chronic low back pain, developing gradually over a period of years, may be indicative of arthritis. Pain in the back during later afternoon and evening hours only may be due to the emotional tension and stress that frequently build up during the day and, in the process, build up muscle tension that may lead to back pain.

We could go on almost indefinitely, but you get the point—the information obtained in a medical history is just as important as any diagnostic test in helping the doctor identify the cause of your back pain! Answer all questions as completely and thoroughly as possible. Do not assume any fact to be too minor or irrelevant. It is not an infrequent occurrence that the physical examination and numerous sophisticated diagnostic tests performed on most back victims ultimately serve only to verify a strongly suspected diagnosis first made by the doctor while obtaining a thorough medical history. The "Pain Evaluation: Patient Form medical history used at our centers is shown in Table 5-1. (See page 80)

PHYSICAL EXAMINATION

The next step in a medical evaluation is the physical examination. When examining the patient with back pain, the doctor approaches the examination in an orderly fashion. Most physical examinations for back pain can be considered as consisting of three components: (1) systemic, (2) functional, and (3) neurological. Since every doctor is an individual with a unique style of practice and the potential checks and balances of a physical examination are almost limitless, we will confine our discussion to the basics of the physical examination procedure. In addition, most doctors recognize that the patient is a whole person who happens to have a bad back and is not just a spine in isolation. Do not be surprised if your physical examination is far more comprehensive than the essentials discussed here.

Systemic Examination

The systemic examination refers to the body as a composite whole or "system" rather than any particular part of the body. This thinking is similar to considering an automobile as a system of transportation rather than as isolated parts such as the brake system, the transmission, or the radiator system. There are several systemic diseases that produce symptoms of back pain that should be investigated during the physical examination. For example, an examination of the abdomen may reveal evidence suggesting that an aortic aneurysm (abnormal swelling of the main trunk of the arterial system of the body) may be producing insufficient blood flow to the vessels in the low back. Insufficient vascular blood flow to the legs or feet may result in a slight limp, which, in turn, disturbs the physical balance of the spine and results in postural low back pain.

A pelvic and rectal examination may also be part of a thorough systemic evaluation. For women with back discomfort, a pelvic exam may reveal a number of potential gynecologic causes of low back pain, including endometriosis, pelvic inflammatory disease, pelvic congestion, and adenomyosis.

Once a review of the body as a complete system has been accomplished, the doctor narrows the scope of investigation to a functional examination of the spine and its associated parts.

Functional Examination

A functional examination can be defined as an assessment of the functioning and impairment or limitation of the spine and its associated body parts. Many physicians will start this part of the physical examination by asking you to remove your clothing and to assume a standing position. The first phase is observation of body posture, outline, spinal contour, pelvic symmetry, leg length, and the inclination of the head, neck, and shoulder levels. Even in this age of sophisticated diagnostic test procedures, the legendary value of educated observation should not be discounted. Many observable postural and mechanical disorders can result in persistent and troublesome back pain.

You may be asked next to participate in a series of exertional activities, all of which provide information about your back problem. Forward flexion is measured by how far the fingers come to the floor when, in a standing position, you "lock your knees and bend at the waist." Extension is just the opposite—how far you can bend backward. Lateral flexion is measured by how far you can slide a hand down the outside of your thigh toward the knee. All of these activities give the doctor information about any limitations of motion you may have in the spine.

You may then be asked to walk toward the doctor on your heels and away on your toes. You may feel a bit foolish and awkward, but this activity provides valuable information about lumbar and sacral muscle and nerve damage.

The next stage is to lie down on the examining table while the doctor presses on your stomach in search of any abdominal mass. Warning—this may tickle a bit! Your pulse may also be checked in both arms and legs to insure proper functioning. Leg lengths are then measured since previously unnoticed discrepancies of as little as 1.5 centimeters may be sufficient to produce postural back strain. Thigh and calf circumference measurements may also be taken. Thigh or calf atrophy (lost tissue mass) can indicate the interruption of specific nerve supplies from the spine to the legs.

While you are on your back, the ankles, feet, knees, and hips are twisted, turned, pushed, and pulled to determine any limitation of motion or production of pain. In addition, the straight-leg-raise test is usually performed. As can be seen in Figure 5-1, this test involves actively or passively raising the leg as high as possible with the knee extended or "locked." If you feel a pulling tightness in the back of the knee and leg, there is little cause for concern. This sensation suggests tightness of the hamstring muscles that run from the lower buttocks to below the knees and may indicate that you are not properly conditioned, but this is not what the examiner is looking for. A straight-leg-raise test that elicits sharp radiating pain may suggest disk herniation. The test may also be performed as you sit on the side of the examining table.

NEUROLOGICAL EXAMINATION

Neurological examination involves the investigation of nerve functioning in various areas of the body, all of which provide additional information about the cause of back pain. The examination may begin by checking to see if there is any damage to the spinal cord. The examiner will usually take the blunt end of a reflex hammer and stroke the soles of both feet. If the spinal cord is functioning properly, your reflexes may make your toes curl down.

If you have experienced numbness or tingling sensations in either leg, the doctor may take a small pin and lightly touch various areas along the leg. This investigation indicates whether pain or

STRAIGHT LEG RAISE TEST

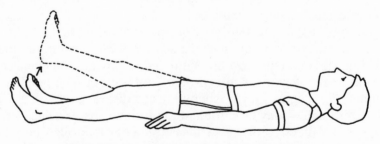

Figure 5-1—The straight-leg-raise test is often part of the medical evaluation of low back pain.

numbness follows a known dermatone pattern. (A dermatone is a segment of skin area supplied by specific spinal nerves.) As can be seen in Figure 5-2, pain or numbness in the big or great toe, for example, can suggest problems with the fifth lumbar nerve since this nerve supplies the area across the skin down to the great toe.

Knee jerk reflexes will also be checked while you are in the sitting position and ankle jerks checked with you kneeling on a chair or in the prone position with knees flexed. Absence or decrease of the knee jerk reflex suggests damage to the fourth lumbar nerve, while absence or decrease in the ankle jerk reflex suggests possible impairment of the first sacral nerve.

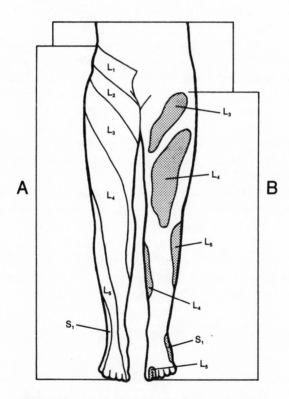

Figure 5-2—Pain, numbness, or other sensation along a dermatome pattern provides information to the examiners and is an important part of the diagnostic evaluation.

LABORATORY TESTS

Although blood and urine laboratory tests are not generally considered to be as beneficial in the diagnosis of low back pain as the history and physical examination, they may provide helpful ancillary information or confirm a doctor's suspicion.

White blood cell count and differential suggest the likelihood of infection of malignancy. The white blood cell count is normal in the great majority of victims of back pain.

Erthrocyte sedimentation rate is a nonspecific but often useful blood screening test to rule out widespread disease and inflammation as the cause of back pain. Unfortunately the erthrocyte sedimentation rate (ESR) may be increased by any infection, even those commonly found in the respiratory or urinary tract. If an initial ESR is elevated, your doctor will probably repeat the study after the infection has subsided before undertaking more extensive testing.

Blood calcium and phosphorus levels are performed on blood samples and give information regarding the structure of bone within the body. When rapid changes occur in the structure of bone, calcium, phosphorus, and other enzymes increase in the blood. This increase reflects the reaction of bone to several types of bone-forming or bone-destroying cancers and a variety of other diseases affecting bone. Laboratory tests that show that these chemicals exist at normal levels will help rule out the possibility of cancer or other diseases as the cause of back pain.

Rheumatoid factor is a laboratory test that may help rule out the possibility of rheumatoid arthritis or some related condition as the cause of the pain. Unfortunately this test is accurate only 75—80 percent of the time and some experts argue that it is useless given these inaccuracies and the fact that rheumatoid arthritis seldom involves the lumbar spine. The test is still used by many doctors, but only in conjunction with a thorough history and physical examination.

X-RAYS

Almost everyone has had an x-ray taken at some time—at the dentist's office, as part of an annual physical examination, or at the doctor's office or hospital because of medical problems. The x-ray has been around a long time and has become a trusted aid in medical diagnosis. But there are a number of misconceptions about x-rays, particularly where the back is concerned.

The greatest misconception surrounds the question of what x-rays show and what they do not show. To understand better the value and limitations of x-rays, keep in mind that they are not photographs or pictures, but are shadows. And just as any individual's overall shadow does not show what he or she looks like, so an x-ray may not directly indicate what is going on in the back. An x-ray of your back shows the shadows cast by the bones of your spine and by the other parts of your body as the rays pass through, or fail to pass through, these structures.

To complicate things further, consider that x-rays are essentially photographic negatives. Try an experiment. Take the negative of a favorite snapshot and hold it to the light. Had you not previously seen the finished photographic print, could you discern any significant detail from the negative? The bones of your spine absorb the x-ray and therefore appear white on the film negative, while other body parts, such as internal organs and muscles, allow much of the x-ray beam to pass through and produce darker areas on film. Reading an x-ray therefore is like trying to "read" the intricate characteristics of an individual's silhouette—a difficult task at best!

An x-ray *cannot* show nerves or disks (except as dark spaces beside lighter shaded bone), muscles, muscle spasm, or, of course, pain. X-ray *can* show bone and bone fractures, bone wear and tear, curvature of the spine (scoliosis), slipped vertebrae (spondylolisthesis), and defective vertebrae (spondylolysis). As an adjunct to a thorough medical history and physical examination, x-rays are relatively safe, are painless, and can often provide valuable information to substantiate or rule out suspected causes of back pain.

SPECIAL TESTS

An initial medical examination for your problem of back pain may conclude with a comprehensive medical history, physical examination, and possibly x-rays of the spine. In most cases your doctor can accurately diagnose the cause of your pain with this information at hand. Treatment will likely be conservative (Chapter 6) since 80 percent or more of all back pain disorders adequately heal in time.

For the 20 percent or so who do not enjoy pain relief as a result of several weeks or months of conservative therapy, the scenario can be quite different. If you are an unfortunate victim of chronic back pain, the chances are excellent that you have been, or eventually will be, faced with a need for more extensive and expensive diagnostic evaluations.

Myelogram

The myelogram is a relatively safe, special x-ray examination of the spinal cord and canal that can help a surgeon diagnose a disk problem, spinal tumor, or spinal abscess. The procedure is normally done in a hospital and, most often, requires that you stay overnight.

Since regular x-rays give only a picture of bone, a special dye that shows up on x-ray must be used in a myelogram. The doctor first withdraws a small portion of the fluid that fills the spinal canal and replaces it with special dye. This is done by carefully injecting a small needle into the lower back to the spinal canal. You may initially feel a stinging sensation followed by a feeling of pressure. Once the dye has been injected, a series of x-ray films are taken. You may be asked to assume different positions or to tilt your head downward. You also may be tilted downward by the examination table, which can be mildly uncomfortable. The tilting motion allows the dye to flow slowly up and down the spine as it fills the space surrounding each spinal nerve. The fluid appears white on x-rays, while any obstruction from protruding disk or tumors show up as dark blotches. The entire procedure usually lasts from 30 to 60 minutes. You may have a headache afterward, but this usually disappears within 24 hours if you follow your doctor's orders to rest flat in bed.

Whether or not to undergo a myelogram should be cautiously considered. Most authorities agree that the test has only an 80–85 percent rate of accuracy. In addition, a small percentage of back pain victims complain that their pain increases following the myelogram. Finally, there is an extremely small but potential risk of paralysis with the procedure. Because of the above, most medical experts today do not consider myelography a routine diagnostic tool, except in cases where a cause for back pain cannot be determined by less invasive forms of testing or where it is required in preparation for surgery. As a general rule, most back surgeons agree that if you are not willing to have surgery, there is little need to undergo a myelogram.

Computerized Tomography

Whether we call them CT (computerized tomography) or CAT (computer-assisted or computerized axial tomography) scans, this technology, which harnesses the power of the computer to the technique of x-raying cross sections of the body, has generated perhaps the most interest of any diagnostic tool developed in the past half-century.

The CT scanner takes a rapid-sequence series of x-ray exposures with a sweeping beam of parallel rays rotating about a longitudinal axis. The finished image is very much like viewing slices of a tomato. Whereas regular x-rays might produce an image of the tomato as a single unit, the CT scanner produces images similar to slicing the tomato into dozens of slices or sections. This allows the diagnostician to view cross sections of your back and examine areas of your spine never before visible. The computer assists by detecting subtle differences between "slices" that are too minor for the human eye to observe. In practical terms this means that the CT scanner can take pictures of soft tissue, nerves, membranes surrounding nerves, and even the internal structure of the spinal cord itself.

Many in the field believe that the CT scanner will ultimately make the myelogram obsolete in the diagnosis of difficult back pain. Certainly the information obtained from CT far outweighs the diagnostic capability of myelography. In addition, myelography is an invasive technique that causes a degree of pain and carries some element of serious risk, whereas CT is virtually risk-free as the patient simply rests on a table that moves him or her through a circular x-ray ring. Finally, CT has proved more cost effective than myelography since we can undergo the procedure as an outpatient. Recovery time following a CT scan is only as long as it takes the patient to dress and walk to the car to go home.

Electromyography

Electromyography (EMG) is a technique of measuring the reaction of a muscle when it is stimulated by a nerve. Suppose, for instance, that not only do you have back pain, but your leg is painful and weak. By inserting extremely fine needles into muscle at several points in the back and along the leg (depending on which muscles are being tested), the examiner can determine whether your muscular contraction and nerve impulses are normal or abnormal. If the recording in your leg is normal, the examiner can conclude that any damage is located at a higher level, such as nerve entrapment or impingement at the spine. The EMG test is uncomfortable, but not really painful, and is quite safe.

Thermography

Thermography is a noninvasive, painless test designed to measure the temperature of the skin over a painful body area. The test is based on the theory that where there is inflammation there will be increased heat on the surface of the skin, created by an increased concentration of blood. For example, in a normal subject the same areas on both the left and right sides of the body should emit the same amount of heat. However, in various painful disorders, temperature differences can be detected on the pictures of a thermogram. Acute or recent pain is usually detected as a "hot" area, whereas chronic or long-lasting pain shows up as a "cold" area. A special photograph shows "hot" and "cold" areas of the body by color differences.

Thermography has long been used to diagnose abnormalities of the female breast, including cancer, but it has only recently been employed in the physical diagnosis of pain states. While the test is painless and safe, most experts agree that additional controlled scientific investigation substantiating the accuracy of thermography will be required before this test is fully accepted as an effective diagnostic procedure for back pain.

Psychological Testing

Highly sophisticated technological advances are extremely important in the diagnosis of back pain, but they address only the *physical* component of pain. Since many *psychological* variables naturally enter into our interpretation of and response to back pain, psychological testing has increasingly become utilized as an adjunct to physical diagnostic procedures. If your doctor requests that you see a clinical psychologist for testing, do not be alarmed. Rather than thinking you are "crazy" or that the pain is "all in your head," your physician is simply attempting to provide the most comprehensive diagnostic work-up possible. Psychological testing provides information about your pain problem in the same way that myelograms, x-rays, CT scans, and electromyography provide information. Pain has both physical and psychological components, and only with the availability of all relevant information can your doctor most accurately diagnose your discomfort and best provide for your treatment.

The most widely used psychological test in the evaluation of back pain is the Minnesota Multiphasic Personality Inventory, better known as the MMPI. This inventory is a 400- or 566-item test (depending on the form used) consisting of a wide variety of questions that require true or false answers. Your responses to the questions are tabulated in a profile that is interpreted by a clinical psychologist in much the same manner that an x-ray is interpreted by a Radiologist or other physician. Various personality traits are identified by the MMPI can provide useful information, such as the role of psychological variables in pain complaints, which patients are most likely to benefit from surgery, and the degree of depression and/or anxiety that the patient is experiencing as a result of pain. As more and more physicians learn the value of psychological testing as an adjunct to physical diagnostic procedures, the use of psychological evaluations is becoming increasingly popular as a routine part of a comprehensive diagnostic work-up.

In 1978 Dr. Nelson Hendler and his colleagues at the Johns Hopkins Hospital, Baltimore, designed a screening test for use with individuals suffering chronic back pain. Questions were formulated after conducting psychological evaluations of over 600 patients treated at a chronic pain treatment center. The test was refined on the basis of how these different groups of patients responded to a series of questions regarding their pain experience and history, and significant related matters such as work, sexual activity, use of medications, and thoughts of suicide. Depending on each patient's score, he or she will fall into one of the three diagnostic categories:

Type I. This category describes individuals who show a normal response to chronic pain. If an operation is indicated, the patient will probably respond well to surgery and is usually willing to participate in all modalities of therapy, including exercise and psychotherapy.

Type II. This category describes individuals who may be considered "exaggerating pain patients." Surgery or other intervention procedures may be recommended with caution since many Type II patients do not respond well to surgery. Type II patients have found a use for chronic pain. The most effective mode of treatment is from a chronic pain center with an emphasis on attitude change toward the pain.

Type III. This category describes individuals who should receive care from a clinical psychologist or psychiatrist. This category describes the type of personality that freely admits to a great many prepain problems and shows considerable difficulty coping with the chronic pain now experienced. Surgery or other intervention should not be carried out without prior approval of a psychological/psychiatric consultation.

If you are interested in knowing how your chronic back pain affects you and how you handle your pain, spend about ten minutes completing the following screening test. You should remember that the test is designed to screen patients for appropriate treatment decisions and is only one of many components involved in making a diagnosis. Do not take the results of this test out of context! It is presented only for your interest.

HENDLER TEN-MINUTE SCREENING TEST FOR CHRONIC BACK PAIN PATIENTS*

Instructions

The following test should take you about ten minutes to complete. For each question choose the statement that most closely applies to you, and mark down the number of points you receive on a separate sheet of paper. This test is specifically designed for back pain patients and may not accurately reflect responses to other types of pain.

    I. How did the pain that you now experience occur?
        (a) Sudden onset with accident of definable event   0
        (b) Slow, progressive onset without acute exacerbation   1
        (c) Slow, progressive onset with acute exacerbation without accident or event   2
        (d) Sudden onset without an accident or definable event   3

*Test copyright 1979 by Nelson Hendler, M.D., M.S. Reprinted by permission.

II. Where do you experience the pain?
- (a) One site, specific, well defined, consistent with anatomical distribution   0
- (b) More than one site, each well defined and consistent with anatomical distribution   1
- (c) One site, inconsistent with anatomical considerstions or not well defined   2
- (d) Vague description, more than one site, of which one is inconsistent with anatomical considerations, or not well defined or anatomically explainable   3

III. Do you ever have trouble falling asleep at night or are you ever awakened from sleep?

(If the answer is "no," score three points and go to question IV.
If the answer is "yes," proceed.)

IIIA. What keeps you from falling asleep, or what awakens you from sleep?
- (a) Trouble falling asleep every night due to pain   0
- (b) Trouble falling asleep due to pain more than three times a week   1
- (c) Trouble falling asleep due to pain less than three times per week   2
- (d) No trouble falling asleep due to pain   3
- (e) Trouble falling asleep which is not related to pain   4

IIIB.
- (a) Awakened by pain every night   0
- (b) Awakened from sleep by pain more than three times a week   1
- (c) Not awakened from sleep by pain more than twice a week   2
- (d) Not awakened from sleep by pain   3
- (e) Restless sleep, or early morning awakening with or without being able to return to sleep, both unrelated to pain   4

IV. Does weather have any effect on your pain?
- (a) Burning; or sharp, shooting pain; or pins and needles; or coldness; or numbness   0
- (b) Dull, aching pain, with occasional sharp shooting pains not helped by heat   1
- (c) Spasm-type pain, tension-type pain, or numbness over the area, relieved by massage or heat   2
- (d) Nagging or bothersome pain   3
- (e) Excruciating, overwhelming, or unbearable pain, relieved by massage or heat   4

VI. How frequently do you have pain?
- (a) The pain is constant   0
- (b) The pain is nearly constant, occurring 50–80 percent of the time   1
- (c) The pain is intermittent, occurring 25–50 percent of the time   2
- (d) The pain is only occasionally present, occurring less than 25 percent of the time   3

VII. What medications have you used in the past month?
- (a) No medications at all   0
- (b) Use of nonnarcotic pain relievers or mild tranquilizers or antidepressants   1
- (c) Less than three-times-a-week use of a narcotic sleeping pill, or tranquilizer   2
- (d) Greater than four-times-a-week use of narcotic, sleeping pill, or tranquilizer   3

VIII. Does movement or position have any effect on the pain?
  (a) The pain is unrelieved by position change or rest, and there have been previous operations for the pain   0
  (b) The pain is worsened by use, standing, or walking, and is relieved by lying down or resting the part   1
  (c) Position change and use have variable effects on the pain   2
  (d) The pain is not altered by use or position by use or position change, and there have been no previous operations for the pain   3

IX. What hobbies do you have, and can you still participate in them?
  (a) Unable to participate in any hobbies that were formerly enjoyed   0
  (b) Reduced number of hobbies or activities relating to a hobby   1
  (c) Still able to participate in hobbies but with some discomforts   2
  (d) Participate in hobbies as before   3

X. How frequently did you have sex and orgasms before the pain and how frequently do you have sex and orgasms now?
  (a1) Sexual contact, prior to pain, three to four times a week, with no difficulty with orgasm; now sexual contact is 50 percent or less than previously, and coitus is interrupted by pain   0
  (a2) (For people over 45) Sexual contact twice a week with a 50 percent reduction in frequency since the pain   0
  (a3) (For people over 65) Sexual contact once a week, with a reduction in frequency of coitus since the onset of pain   0
  (b) Prepain adjustment as defined above (a1–a3) with no difficulty with orgasm; now loss of interest in sex and/or difficulty with orgasm or erection   1
  (c) No change in sexual activity now as opposed to before the onset of pain   2
  (d) Unable to have sexual contact since the onset of pain, and difficulty with orgasm or erection prior to the pain   3
  (e) No sexual contact prior to the pain, or absence of orgasm prior to the pain   4

XI. Are you still working or doing your household chores?
  (a) Working every day at the same prepain job or same level of household duties   0
  (b) Working every day but the job is not the same as prepain job, with reduced responsibility or physical activity   1
  (c) Working sporadically or doing a reduced amount of household chores   2
  (d) Not working at all or all household chores are now performed by others   3

XII. What is your income now compared with before your injury or the onset of pain, and what are your sources of income?
  (a) Any one of the following answers scores   0
    1. Experiencing financial difficulty with family income 50 percent or less than previously
    2. Was retired and is still retired
    3. Patient is still working and is not having financial difficulties
  (b) Experiencing financial difficulty with family income only 50–75 percent of the prepain income   1
  (c) Patient unable to work, and receives some compensation so that the family income is at least 75 percent of the prepain income   2

(d) Patient unable to work and receives no compensation but the spouse works and family income is still 75 percent of the prepain income   3

(e) Patient doesn't work, yet the income from disability or other compensation sources is 80 percent or more of gross pay before the pain; the spouse does not work   4

XIII. Are you suing anyone, or is anyone suing you, or do you have an attorney helping you with compensation or disability payments?

(a) No suit pending, and do not have an attorney   0
(b) Litigation is pending, but is not related to the pain   1
(c) The patient is being sued as the result of an accident   2
(d) Litigation is pending or worker's compensation case with a lawyer   3

XIV. If you had three wishes for anything in the world, what would you wish for?

(a) "Get rid of the pain" is the only wish   0
(b) "Get rid of the pain" is one of the three wishes   1
(c) My wishes would be something of a personal nature, such as having more money, having a better relationship with my spouse, or having a bigger house   2
(d) My wishes would be for something like peace in the world, an end to hunger, or something else for others   3

XV. Have you ever been depressed or thought of suicide?

(a) I have been depressed, or I have been depressed in addition to my pain; my depression makes me cry at times and think of suicide   0
(b) Because of the pain, I have been depressed, and I've felt guilty and angry   1
(c) I felt depressed before the pain, or before the pain I suffered a financial or personal loss (death of a friend, family member moved away), and now with the pain here, I also have some depression   2
(d) I don't feel depressed, I don't have crying jags, or I don't feel blue   3
(e) Before the pain I had a history of suicide attempts   4

Point Total

Add up your points and turn back to the description of the three types of pain categories to see how personality variables may be influencing your pain. A score of 18 points or less suggests that you are a Type I personality; 19 to 31 points, a Type II personality; and 32 or more points, a Type III personality.

Remember: This screening device is but one of many techniques, both physical and psychological, that your doctor may use in evaluating your pain. Taken alone, it has little value other than being of interest.

TABLE 5-1
PAIN THERAPY CENTER
Chronic Pain Rehabilitation Program
GREENVILLE GENERAL HOSPITAL
100 MALLARD STREET
Greenville, South Carolina 29601
(803) 242-8088
PAIN EVALUATION: PATIENT FORM

This questionnaire is intended to summarize
information important in the evaluation of pain.

1. Date
2. Name
Last

First

Middle

3. Address
No. Street

City

State

Zip

4. Phone
Area Code

5. Date of Birth
6. Sex: Male ( ) Female ( )
7. Social Security Number—— —— ——
8. Referring Physician
9. Referring Physician's Address
10. Your Religion: (a) Protestant (Give denomination)
                     (b) Catholic ( )
                     (c) Jewish ( )
                     (d) Other (specify)
                     (e) None ( )
11. Ethnic Group: (a) White ( )
                     (b) Black ( )
                     (c) Oriental ( )
                     (d) American Indian ( )
                     (e) Other (specify)
12. Country of Birth:

                     (a) Yourself
                     (b) Mother
                     (c) Father

13. Education: Highest grade of school completed:
        (a) Less than 8th grade ( )
        (b) Completed 8th grade ( )
        (c) Did not complete high school ( )
        (d) Completed high school ( )
        (e) Technical or business school ( )
        (f) Some College ( )
        (g) Completed college ( )
        (h) Graduate or professional school ( )

14. Do you (check all that apply):
        (a) Live alone ( )
        (b) With Spouse ( )
        (c) With children ( )
        (d) With others (roommate, etc.) ( )
        (e) With brothers and/or sisters ( )
        (f) With other relatives (specify)

15. Current Marital Status:
        (a) Married ( ) How long?
        (b) Divorced ( ) How long?
        (c) Separated ( ) How long?
        (d) Single - Never married ( )
        (e) Widowed ( ) How long?

16. If married, how would you describe your marriage?
        (a) Very satisfactory ( )
        (b) Satisfactory ( )
        (c) Tolerable ( )
        (d) Intolerable ( )

17. Causes of marital problems and conflicts (check all that apply):
        (a) Money ( )
        (b) Children ( )
        (c) Parents and/or in-laws ( )
        (d) Work situation ( )
        (e) Personality differences ( )
        (f) Sexual problems ( )
        (g) Physical illnesses ( )
        (h) Religion ( )
        (i) My pain ( )

18. Weekly family income from all sources:
        (a) Less than $100 ( )
        (b) $101 - $200 ( )
        (c) $201 - $300 ( )
        (d) $301 - $400 ( )
        (e) Over $401 ( )

19. Number of individuals supported on family income:

20. Check all sources of income:
        (a) Salary ( )
        (b) Retirement ( )
        (c) Pension ( )
        (d) Social Security ( )
        (e) Personal Disability Insurance ( )
        (f) Investments ( )
        (g) Compensation ( )
        (h) Social Security Disability ( )
        (i) Other (describe)

21. If married, what is your spouse's occupation? (Be specific)

The following questions relate to your employment which includes work as a housewife. Please answer all questions that apply to you:

(1) At what age did you begin working?

(2) How many jobs have you had since you first began working?

(3) What is your specific occupation (include housewife) and briefly describe what you do.

(4) Are you presently employed: Full-time ( ) Part-time ( ) Housewife ( )
     If employed how long?

5. If you are unemployed or employed part-time, is this due to your present pain condition? No ( ) Yes ( )

(6) How long have you been working in your last job?
     If unemployed, retired or disabled, how long?

(7) Do you enjoy your work? (Include housewife):
     (a) All the time ( )
     (b) Most of the time ( )
     (c) Some of the time ( )
     (d) Rarely or not at all ( )

(8) Does your work provide you with a feeling of satisfaction? (Include housewife):
     (a) All of the time ( )
     (b) Most of the time ( )
     (c) Some of the time ( )
     (d) Rarely or not at all ( )

(9) In general, before your injury, did your employer treat you fairly?
     Yes ( )   No ( )

23. If your present pain condition was caused by your job or occurred while on the job or was due to an accident, please answer the following:
     (1) Was your employer helpful and understanding of your problem?
          Yes ( )   No ( )
     2(2) Do you believe he has been fair in his treatment of you since you have been sick/injured?
          Yes ( )   No ( )
     (3) Have you received compensation (money) for your injury?
          Yes ( )   No ( )
     (4) If you have received compensation, do you feel it has been adequate?
          Yes ( )   No ( )
     (5) Are you bringing suit (suing) because of your injury?
          Yes ( )   No ( )
     (6) Have you already had to sue to get compensation?
          Yes ( )   No ( )
     (7) Have you tried to return to work?
          Yes ( )   No ( )
     (8) Did your employer allow you to return?
          Yes ( )   No ( )
     (9) Do you think you can work at your regular job?
          (a) Full time ( )
          (b) Part-time ( )
          (c) Not at all ( )
     (10) Compared to your ability to do your job before your injury:
          (a) Can you now do as much as before?
          (b) Do somewhat less than before?
          (c) Do much less than before?
          (d) Can't do the job at all?

24. Comparing yourself before you had pain with your present condition, please answer the questions below:
    (1) My *desire* for social activities:
        (a) Remains about the same as before ( )
        (b) Somewhat less than before ( )
        (c) Very much less than before ( )
        (d) No desire for social activities ( )
    (2) My *ability* to engage in social activities:
        (a) Remains about the same as before ( )
        (b) Is somewhat less than before ( )
        (c) Is very much less than before ( )
        (d) I no longer have the ability ( )
    (3) My *desire* for hobbies and recreational interests:
        (a) Remains about the same as before ( )
        (b) Is somewhat less than before ( )
        (c) Is very much less than before ( )
        (d) No desire for hobbies or recreation ( )
    (4) My *ability* to engage in hobbies and recreational activities:
        (a) Remains about the same as before ( )
        (b) Is somewhat less than before ( )
        (c) Is very much less than before ( )
        (d) I no longer have the ability ( )
    (5) My *desire* for sexual activities:
        (a) Remains about the same as before ( )
        (b) Is somewhat less than before ( )
        (c) Is very much less than before ( )
        (d) No desire for sexual relations ( )
    (6) My *ability* to engage in sexual activities:
        (a) Remains about the same as before ( )
        (b) Is somewhat less than before ( )
        (c) Is very much less than before ( )
        (d) I no longer have the ability ( )
25. Have you ever had psychological or psychiatric treatment or evaluation for any condition or problem? If yes, give condition of most recent treatment
    Yes ( ) Date   No ( )
26. Do you feel you are helpless to change your present condition?
    (a) Never ( )
    (b) Some of the time ( )
    (c) Most of the time ( )
    (d) All of the time ( )
27. Do you feel your present condition is hopeless?
    (a) Never ( )
    (b) Some of the time ( )
    (c) Most of the time ( )
    (d) All of the time ( )
28. Aside from your pain problem, are you frequently ill?
    Yes ( )   No ( )
29. Are you frequently confined to bed because of poor health, other than because of pain?
    Yes ( )   No ( )
30. Do others consider you a sickly person?
    Yes ( )   No ( )
31. Do you consider yourself to be a sickly person?
    Yes ( )   No ( )
32. Do you come from a sickly family?
    Yes ( )   No ( )

33. Was any member of your family disabled because of a pain problem?
Yes ( )   No ( )
34. Does it seem that suffering is your way of life?
    (a) Never ( )
    (b) Sometimes ( )
    (c) Most of the time ( )
    (d) Always feel that way ( )
35. Are you often miserable and unhappy? Yes ( ) No ( )
    (a) Is your appetite: Good ( ) Poor ( )
    (b) Do you have crying spells or feel like it? Yes ( ) No ( )
    (c) Are you more irritable than usual? Yes ( ) No ( )
36. The following frequently increase (↑) or decrease (↓) chronic pain. Please mark ↑ for increase or ↓ for decrease to all of the following that apply to you and your pain:

Stimulants (coffee, etc.)	——	Lying down	——
Liquor	——	Sitting	——
Eating	——	Driving	——
Heat	——	Distraction (T.V.,etc.)	——
Cold	——	Urinating	——
Dampness	——	Bowel movement	——
Weather Change	——	Tension	——
Massage, vibrator	——	Bright lights	——
Pressure	——	Loud noises	——
Movement	——	Going to work	——
Standing	——	Sexual activity	——
Bending	——	Sneezing	——
Mild exercise	——	Coughing	——

37. Do you think your pain is due to something more serious or different from what your doctors have told you?
Yes ( )   No ( )
What do you think is the cause?

38. Since your pain began, which of the following people have you seen for treatment and pain relief?

     1. Acupuncturist ( )
     2. Allergist ( )
     3. Anesthesiologist ( )
     4. Cardiologist ( )
     5. Chiropractor ( )
     6. Clergyman ( )
     7. Dentist ( )
     8. Dermatologist ( )
     9. Otorhinolaryngologist ( ) (ear, nose and throat)
    10. Endocrinologist ( )
    11. Faith healer ( )
    12. General or family doctor ( )
    13. Gynecologist/Obstetrician ( )
    14. Hypnotist ( )
    15. Internal Medicine ( )
    16. Neurologist ( )
    17. Neurosurgeon ( )
    18. Opthalmologist (eyes) ( )
    19. Orthopedist (bones & joints) ( )
    20. Osteopath ( )
    21. Plastic Surgeon ( )
    22. Proctologist ( )
    23. Psychiatrist ( )
    24. Psychologist ( )
    25. Radiologist ( )
    26. Surgeon (general) ( )
    27. Physiatrist ( )
    28. Others (specify)

39. Have doctors ever suggested that your pain was imaginary or "all in your head"?
Yes ( )   No ( )
40. Have any doctors or nurses ever acted as if they thought you were faking?
Yes ( )   No ( )
41. How did your pain begin?
    (a) Accident at work ( )
    (b) Accident at home ( )

    (c) Other accident ( )
    (d) At work but not accident ( )
    (e) Following surgery ( )
    (f) Following illness ( )
    (g) Pain just began one day ( )
    (h) Other reasons
42. Please describe briefly your answer to question 41.

43. When did you first experience the pain for which you are now seeking help?
    Date
44. In what parts of the body did the pain begin? (Name all parts)

45. Is the Pain:
    (a) Rarely present ( )
    (b) Only occurs under certain conditions ( )
    (c) Frequently present ( )
    (d) Usually present ( )
    (e) Always present ( )
46. Describe your answer to Question Number 45.

47. Is the *intensity* of your pain always the same or is it sometimes worse?
    Same ( )   Worse ( )
48. Describe your answer to Question Number 47.

49. The following words describe degrees of pain severity:
    1 = Mild   3 = Fairly Severe   5 = unberable,
    2 = Uncomfortable   4 = Very severe, horrible   excruciating
    Please write the number of the word which best describes:
    (a) Your pain as it usually feels ——
    (b) Your pain *right now* ——
    (c) Your pain at its *worse* ——
    (d) Your pain when it hurts *least* ——
    (e) The *worst* toothache you ever had ——
    (f) The *worst* headache you ever had ——
    (g) The *worst* stomachache you ever had ——
    (h) The *worst* sunburn you ever had ——
    (i) The *worst* insect bite you ever had ——
50. Do you have trouble falling asleep?
    (a) Never ( )
    (b) Sometimes ( )
    (c) Usually ( )
    (d) Always ( )
51. Do you take medicine to help you sleep?
    (a) Never ( )
    (b) Sometimes ( )
    (c) Usually ( )
    (d) Always ( )
    What is the name of the medicine?
52. Does the pain frequently wake you at night?
    Yes ( )   No ( )
    If yes, how many times on an average night?

When it does wake you up, what do you usually do?
(a) Empty bladder ( )
(b) Take medication ( )
(c) Sit up for awhile ( )
(d) Other (describe)

53. What does your husband or wife do when you wake up at night? (Do not just say "nothing"—be specific.)

54. What activities bring on the pain or make the pain worse?

55. About how long after beginning this activity does it take for the pain to begin or become worse?

56. Does the pain stop if you quit doing these activities?

57. How many times a day do you have to stop what you are doing because of the pain?

58. How many times a day do you have to lie down because of the pain?
59. Do you have days when the pain is so bad that you stay in bed?
Yes ( )   No ( )
How often does this happen?
60. If I were there when you were in pain, what would I see and hear? How do others around you know when you are in pain? (Describe fully.)

61. When you are in pain, what does your husband or wife do?

62. Have you ever been operated on for your pain?
(a) Never ( )
(b) Once ( )
(c) Twice ( )
(d) Three times ( )
(e) Four times ( )
(f) Five times ( )
(g) More than five times ( )
(1) Date of last operation
(2) Did any operation bring relief from the pain? Yes ( )   No ( )
(3) What is the longest period of relief after an operation?
63. Have you ever had nerve blocks (injections) for the pain?
Yes ( )   No ( )
If yes, how many?
64. Do you take medicine for relief of your pain? Yes ( ) No ( )
Is it medicine that your doctor ordered? Yes ( ) No ( )
Is it medicine that you decided to take yourself? Yes ( ) No ( )
65. What medicines are you *now* taking for pain and how often do you take each one?

Pain Medicine	Dose	Frequency	Date Started
1.			
2.			
3.			
4.			
5.			
6.			
7.			

66. What other medicines do you take for conditions other than pain?
    Medication   Dose   Frequency   Date Started
    1.
    2.
    3.
    4.
67. How effective is the pain medication you take?
    (a) Always takes pain away ( )
    (b) Always makes pain less ( )
    (c) Usually takes pain away ( )
    (d) Usually makes pain less ( )
    (e) Frequently takes pain away ( )
    (f) Frequently makes pain less ( )
    (g) No effect at all ( )
68. What is the *longest* time that your medicine relieves your pain?
69. If you are *not* working now and had no pain problem, would you plan to go back to work?
    Yes ( )   No ( )
    To the same job you had before your injury?
    Yes ( )   No ( )
70. If you could have *any* job, what would you really like to do?

71. What do you want from the Pain Program—be as specific as you can.

72. What do you expect from treatment—be as specific as you can.

73. Do you feel that the doctors who have treated you for your pain have been sympathetic and understanding?
    (a) Very sympathetic ( )
    (b) Somewhat sympathetic ( )
    (c) Hardly sympathetic ( )
    (d) Not at all sympathetic ( )
74. How would you rate your overall satisfaction with the care and treatment you have received for your pain so far?
    (a) Very satisfied ( )
    (b) Somewhat satisfied ( )
    (c) Barely satisfied ( )
    (d) Dissatisfied ( )
    (e) Very dissatisfied ( )
75. If your treatment here does not bring you relief, do you think you will try somewhere else?
    Yes ( )   No ( )

6

CONSERVATIVE TREATMENT

After a thorough physical examination with special attention to your back, your doctor will next prescribe some type of treatment aimed at reducing your distress. The treatment alternatives are practically endless and the remainder of this book is devoted to a discussion of the advantages and disadvantages of many different treatments, including the TOLLISON PROGRAM FOR DAILY BACK PAIN MANAGEMENT.

The first treatment approach prescribed by most doctors is likely to be conservative in nature. This is not without good reason, even though many back pain victims protest the time-consuming conservative approach in favor of a more aggressive approach such as surgery. These individuals believe that surgery and aggressive treatments will hasten pain relief, but unfortunately this is not always the case. Conservative treatment is without doubt the most logical approach for the following reasons. First, 90 percent of all back pain victims will experience gradual pain relief with conservative treatment alone. Since the statistical odds are heavily in favor of relief through conservative treatment, it hardly makes sense to subject yourself to the risks, side effects, and dangers of surgery and powerful medications. Second, there is growing evidence that surgery to relieve pain is unsuccessful in over 50 percent of the cases. This does not mean that there is no useful place for back surgery. There are instances when surgery is required to stop deteriorating back problems but these are few. In the great majority of cases, surgery has simply not proved as effective as conservative treatment in reducing the misery of a painful back.

Conservative treatment generally takes time and requires that you assume responsibility for managing your back pain. The results are usually well worth the trouble.

BED REST

The first instruction you are likely to be given is to go home and go to bed. Indeed, most physicians were well trained in the idea that back pain should be treated with bed rest and muscle relaxant medication. How long you are told to stay in bed depends on the physician and can range from one to six weeks. The theory behind conservative bed rest is simple—staying in bed for several weeks restricts movement, pressure, and strain on the back and allows the injured tissue time to heal. Tranquilizers and muscle relaxants are given to help keep you calm and your muscles relaxed during the time your back takes to heal. Occasionally home traction is also prescribed as it is believed by some health professionals to provide a measure of relief and healing while ensuring that you remain in bed.

Does conservative bed rest work to heal your painful back, reduce the waiting time for pain relief, decrease the incidence of chronic pain, or lessen the frequency of long-term back disability? In my experience the answer in most cases is no!

Coinciding with the training and development of "pain specialists" as a new branch of health care in the past several years has been a reexamination of many traditionally instructed and accepted treatment techniques for pain management. With the increasing attention to pain as a primary disorder, rather than the traditional indirect view of pain as a secondary problem or symptom of some primary disorder, has come a questioning of treatment techniques long accepted as fact. One such reconsideration of the value of conservative bed rest has resulted in a controversy over bed rest versus exercise. The question is this: In the treatment of back pain, which treatment is most effective—bed rest or movement and exercise?

Traditional medical education has long praised the therapeutic value of bed rest in the treatment of back pain, particularly *acute* back pain. However, now pain clinics are widely recommending exercise performed either *passively* with another person, such as a physical therapist, moving your limbs for you, or *actively* on your own. This recommendation not only considers the effects of exercise on the body, but the psychological benefits as well. Joining an exercise class or, better yet, being involved in a supervised exercise program available at many pain clinics gets the sufferer out of the house and, just as important, associating with people. Exercise helps keep your joints limber and flexible while bed rest usually results in a gradual deconditioning of the body and the onset of stiffness, reduced range of joint motion, and increased pain upon movement. In addition, muscle relaxants leave us groggy, fatigued, and feeling washed out. I have trouble understanding the injunction, "Stay in bed and take these muscle relaxants and I'll give you a letter to return to work in three weeks." After three weeks of bed rest and muscle relaxants with resulting joint stiffness, muscle soreness, fatigue, dizziness, and total body deconditioning, who could suddenly return to work and activity, even if the back pain were reduced?

I recall an acute pain episode as part of my own back problem that suddenly brought me to my knees many years ago. It occurred as the result of poor body mechanics when lifting and took place years before I became convinced of the value of movement and exercise. Following my doctor's advice, I stayed in bed for almost a week and swallowed muscle relaxants every four hours as directed. I vividly recall the frustration and irritation of being confined to bed and the horrible nightmares caused by the medication. When I could take it no longer and left the bed, I remember the overall body soreness, stiffness, and pain that did not go away until I had been up and moving about for several days. I knew then that there must be a better way to manage back pain and years later found the treatment regimen that works well for me. Now when I experience the infrequent episodes of acute and severe back pain, I limit myself to one day of bed rest and aspirin rather than muscle relaxants and tranquilizers. The following day I am up and moving around. Though my back will hurt for several days, I am mobile and avoid the irritation, frustration, muscle soreness, joint stiffness, and nightmares associated with bed rest and medications.

Dr. Hans Kraus, a specialist in physical medicine and rehabilitation who treated President John F. Kennedy for his lower back pain, is another strong advocate of exercise. In his book *Sports Injuries*, Dr. Kraus recommends "MECE not RICE." RICE is an acronym for what most physicians recommend for acute strains and sprains: rest, ice, compression, and elevation. MECE stands for movement, ethyl cholride (a cooling spray that acts as a local anesthetic), and elevation. Says Dr. Kraus, "Rest doesn't promote healing—movement does."

Before discarding the idea of bed rest in favor of movement and exercise to manage your back pain, you are cautioned to consult your physician. In numerous places throughout this book, I will remind you that effective back pain management is a partnership effort between patient and physician. Partners consult on all important decisions. There does exist a very small number of back pain problems that would be made worse by movement and exercise, but this number is far smaller than many professionals believe. Discuss your desire to try movement and exercise and explain your reasons. Most physicians will approve your plan and you will have taken a major step toward effective back pain management.

MANIPULATION AND MASSAGE

Sooner or later, many people with chronic back pain will give up on their doctors and turn elsewhere for help. Perhaps it is the fault of the physician, who may keep the sufferer coming back for appointments and do little more than make slight changes in medications. Other physicians either may refuse or do not think to refer the patient to a pain clinic where better management of the pain can be taught. In still other instances, the patient may not want to assume responsibility for the pain or to expend the necessary efforts to manage it effectively and prefers to go "shopping for a cure." These individuals refuse to accept the fact that while chronic back pain is seldom a "curable" problem, it can be managed with little disruption in life-style if the victim is willing to try. Regardless of who is at fault, a percentage of back pain sufferers will reject traditional medical care in favor of exploring alternatives.

One such alternative I call the "shrine syndrome," which is characterized by the pain victim's desire to make a holy pilgrimage to a faraway, expensive, well-known mystical shrine of healing. This syndrome usually starts with the patient's declaration that, "I don't care how much it costs—I want the very best!" Often these "shrines" are part of prestigious medical schools, although others are independent businesses that cater to the pain pilgrim. Regardless of where they are located, the doctors and health professionals involved are likely to see themselves as standing apart and above the main body of health professionals and they take every opportunity to promote the idea that they are "healers" where other, lesser professionals have failed.

These "Meccas of Medical Magic" function in an advantageous, no-lose situation. First, they enjoy a profound placebo effect in that pain victims truly believe they will be helped and, by virtue of this belief, are already helped. Second, in the very slight chance that lasting relief is accomplished, the shrine is credited with yet another miracle performed after other health professionals have failed. Finally, in the frequently occurring event that shrine treatment fails, there is always the excuse that, "If only your doctor had sent you here earlier, we could have helped you." The pain pilgrim generally returns from the pilgimage with the same intensity of pain, financially distraught, and blaming local doctors for the sad situation.

In addition to the "shrine syndrome," other dissatisfied back pain victims may turn to alternative health care practitioners in search of relief. While anyone disenchanted with conventional health care will have no trouble finding a wide variety of promising others, osteopaths, chiropractors, and physical therapists control the domain of "manipulation and massage" and are probably the three most frequently consulted alternative groups.

Osteopaths

Has repeated scientific study confirmed the value of manipulation and massage in the treatment of back pain? Not really, but many health professionals who have clinical experience with manipulative techniques feel they are truly helping patients with back discomfort.

"Manipulation" is a broad rubric for the use of hands in the treatment of patients. The term is often subcategorized according to the grades of force used, ranging from soft tissue massage, to pushing a joint through its entire range of motion, to "back cracking." Each maneuver varies according to the manipulator's particular method, and during a treatment session a variety of techniques will usually be employed.

Osteopaths were the first professionals trained in the art of manipulation and massage. Osteopathy was founded over 100 years ago by A. T. Still in Missouri, who made an extensive study of human anatomy and developed a number of manipulative techniques based on the laws of anatomy, physics, and leverage. His followers grew both in numbers and in skill. In time osteopathic medical schools were founded in Europe and the United States. These early schools differed greatly from conventional allopathic medical schools and osteopaths found themselves at a great disadvantage in competition with better-known, accepted, and organized allopathic medicine. Allopathic physicians earned the "M.D.," or doctor-of-medicine, degree whereas osteopaths earned the "D.O.," or doctor-of-osteopathy degree—and the difference in degrees had far-reaching ramifications. The well-established, richly funded, and politically active American Medical Association (AMA) lobbied to hold their control of health care by efforts to keep osteopaths from being recognized as physicians by the federal government and military, and also by prohibiting their recognition by national insurance companies. Hospitals dependent on allopathic physicians to admit patients were directly or indirectly threatened if consideration was given to allowing osteopaths on the medical staff.

During the many years of political maneuvering, jealousy, lobbying, name calling, and total lack of harmony between the AMA and the American Osteopathic Association, osteopathic schools were quietly shifting and broadening their focus of medical instruction to resemble more closely the education of allopathic physicians. Manipulation was deemphasized and anatomy, physiology, pathology, and pharmacology received added emphasis. Perhaps this philosophical shift was a natural evolution, or perhaps it was based on the philosophy, "If you can't beat them, join them!" Regardless of the reason, the training of allopathic and osteopathic physicians grew increasingly similar until the AMA finally gave up the fight and admitted osteopaths to the association with full rights and equal standing.

Today osteopaths can hardly be distinguished from allopathic physicians. Very few osteopaths continue to rely heavily on spinal manipulation and massage; the majority practice traditional medical care. These days if you visit an osteopath for your back problem, you may receive manipulative treatment, but are more likely to be prescribed the bed rest, medication, electrical therapies, or surgery commonly advised by allopathic physicians.

Chiropractors

As the osteopath moved from emphasizing spinal manipulation and massage toward more conventional medicine, the vacancy was quickly and aggressively filled by the chiropractor. The word "chiropractor" is derived from the Greek words *cheir* and *praklikis* meaning "done by the hand." The approach is based on the philosophy that spinal vertebrae become misaligned or subluxated and thereby exert pressure on spinal nerves, which ultimately leads to illness, disease, and pain. Chiropractic was founded by Dr. Daniel David Palmer who practiced as a "healer." In 1895, Palmer had the opportunity to examine a man who had been deaf for 17 years. The loss of hearing had occurred after the victim had felt something "give" in his back. The story goes that Palmer gave a crude spinal adjustment to what he believed was a misplaced vertebra in the upper spine and the patient's hearing improved. Although many modern chiropractors have incorporated electrical stimulation, diathermy, ultrasound, and a variety of other electrical therapies into their practice, the mainstay of chiropractic remains spinal manipulation or "adjustments." Chiropractic adjustment are hypothesized to realign the spine, thereby relieving pressure on the spinal nerves and restoring the natural nerve function throughout the body. When the spine is properly aligned, the body is supposedly in a natural state of balance or homeostasis and the individual is free from illness, disease, and pain.

If you take your aching back to a chiropractor, this is what you can expect. First, the chiropractor will usually obtain a medical history—Where does your back hurt? How long have you had pain? What makes the pain worse? And so on. This history may also include an evaluation of your nutrition, alcohol and drug intake, work habits, and levels of stress. Next, a hands-on physical examination is usually conducted and your legs, back, arms, and neck may be turned, twisted, pushed, and pulled to determine any limitation in motion in a joint or joints. X-rays of your spine then may be taken, which the chiropractor "reads" to determine which vertebrae are subluxated or misaligned (it should be noted that medical doctors and chiropractors often disagree over the interpretation of x-rays). Finally, treatment is based on manipulation of or "adjustments" to the spine, although some chiropractors also use vitamins, massage, and electrical therapies as part of their treatment.

Chiropractic is the second largest healing art and over 40 million

Americans routinely receive chiropractic treatment. Because of this and major theoretical and philosophical differences, it may come as no surprise that chiropractors and medical doctors have traditionally not been part of a mutual admiration society. But the gap appears to be closing and differences decreasing. Many of organized medicine's criticisms, such as inferior chiropractic training and the chiropractic belief that all illnesses and diseases are caused by nerve impingements in the spine, are being neutralized by the chiropractic profession. In recent years chiropractic colleges have greatly upgraded the student-selection process, educational content, and faculty composition in their schools. Chiropractic students are now taught not only by other chiropractors, but by a scattering of medical doctors and Ph.D.s as well. In addition, courses common in medical education but never before allowed in chiropractic curricula are springing up with increased frequency in chiropractic colleges. Far removed from older pioneers, the newly graduated chiropractor is likely to deemphasize the traditional chiropractic belief of nerve impingement and disease and emphasize the treatment of musculoskeletal disorders and physical therapies. In fact, in recent years the American Chiropractic Association has voted to no longer support the idea that disease, illness, and pain come only from spinal nerve impingements and now recognize a far greater variety of possible causes of physical disorders. Also unlike his or her predecessors, the modern chiropractor seems anxious to refer to medical doctors those problems thought to be caused by underlying pathology. Like the osteopaths before it, modern chiropractic seems to be moving toward conventional medicine.

Can conservative chiropractic treatment help your aching back? The answer depends a great deal on the cause of your back discomfort and the skill of the chiropractor. Pain caused by stiff joints and muscle spasms is more likely to respond to manipulation and massage than other types of back disorders. If you have considered giving chiropractic a trial, why not conduct an informal investigation? See a chiropractor for six visits. At the end of that period, if you are not getting better or if the problem is worse, stop the investigation. If you are feeling better, then continue in treatment.

Physical Therapy

Physical therapy is an important treatment for almost all back pain sufferers. The physical therapist is not a doctor, but a skilled technician who carries out your doctor's orders to exercise tight and painful parts of your body. In treating chronic back pain, physical therapy should involve both treatment and educational components. For example, physical therapists are trained to conduct postural instruction, education in basic anatomy and physiology, instruction in body mechanics, and instruction in stretching, strengthening, and conditioning exercises for back pain victims. In addition, the physical therapist works closely with your doctor to determine if specific "modality" techniques are indicated in your case. Such techniques may include ultrasound, heat, diathermy, TENS, electrical stimulation, hydrotherapy, massage, and, believe it or not, spinal manipulation.

Many physical therapists have borrowed a page from the notebook of early osteopathy and modern chiropractic and are staking their claim to a share of the spinal manipulation business. This broadening of the physical therapist's scope of practice cannot be faulted from an economic point of view since many such therapists are breaking away from salaried hospital positions and going into private practice. There is a great deal of money in spinal manipulation and no one has ever criticized the profession of physical therapy for being economically ignorant or overly charitable. Many of the same medical doctors who have historically criticized osteopathic and chiropractic "spinal manipulation" and "gadget therapy" are now referring a steady stream of back pain victims to physical therapists for much of the same treatment they have argued against. Because of this many individuals are now questioning whether the real concern of organized medicine is the "treatment" or the "practitioner" providing the treatment.

If you and your bad back are referred to physical therapy, this is what you can expect. First, an evaluation will be conducted by a therapist to determine any limitation in joint motion, muscle weakness, and the distribution of your back pain. Treatment will probably center around heat packs applied to the area of pain. Ultrasound or diathermy (deep heating techniques) may also be given, as well as back massages. The treatment will be quite soothing and pleasant but, unfortunately, of very short-term benefit. In the experiences of most of the patients I see, traditional physical therapy modality treatments provide only temporary relief, and before you get home from the therapist's office you are likely in as much pain as before you went. This is particularly true if your back pain is chronic in nature.

The problem, I think, goes back to our earlier discussion of the controversy over bed rest versus exercise. Physical therapists are trained in physical therapy departments that are generally part of medical schools. Since traditional medical education has emphasized rest and recovery for back pain, it follows that physical therapists have been taught to augment this with gentle, pleasant, and soothing treatments such as heat and massage. The plan may sound great but the enormous number of chronic back pain victims evidences the fact that it has not been perfected.

Perhaps physical therapy should emphasize movement, exercise, strenghthening, conditioning, and graduated activity instead. As previously discussed, many health professionals now believe that rather than helping the back pain victim reduce pain and return to a more productive life style, the traditional techniques of treating back discomfort may actually set the stage for developing *chronic* backache.

TRACTION

Traction has been used for years in the treatment of spinal pain. However, practitioners are gradually accepting the idea that traction produces better results with neck problems than with disorders of the lower back. Consequently the use of traction in the treatment of low back pain appears to be decreasing.

The idea behind traction is that if vertebrae pressing on spinal nerves (pinched nerve) can be stretched apart to allow added space for the nerves within their exit canals, then pain should be relieved. Obviously traction is primarily designed for pain resulting from pinched nerves and is generally not prescribed for other types of back pain. While traction can easily stretch the neck and relieve pressure on spinal nerves, the size of the trunk, the bulk of the back muscles, and even the shape of the vertebrae make stretching of the low back extremely difficult.

To be most effective, many practitioners believe that traction should be sustained. For example, depending on the personal beliefs and philosophy of the physician, traction may be continuously applied for one and a half or two hours and then released for a half hour of rest. The amount of weight used in traction is also based on the beliefs and philosophy of the physician and may range from a couple of pounds up to eight or ten pounds of pull on the neck, and considerably more weighted pull if treating the lower back. Milder cases of neck pain can sometimes benefit from intermittent traction applied several times weekly during visits to a physical therapist or other practitioner. For example, I have a physician friend who hangs upside down with his knees over the crossbar of his children's swing set several times each week to relieve his mild but irritating back pain. This modified traction technique may work for my friend, but it is not a recommended treatment!

Like any treatment designed to improve your condition without effecting a cure, traction should relieve your symptoms of pain within the first few treatments. If traction does not reduce your pain, or more important, if it increases your pain, stop treatment and discuss the situation with your doctor.

Some people spend a lot of money on gadgets, including slings, harnesses, pulleys, weights, and other devices advertised to relieve back pain misery. Two of the more novel (and stranger) types are vertical traction and gravity boots.

Vertical traction uses an apparatus that attaches around the chest and leaves you suspended in air in a vertical position. Such units are not inexpensive and considerable effort is required to hang suspended. If your back is already strong and mobile enough to withstand the contortions required to attach the device, some may question whether the treatment is really needed. More significant, and perhaps more dangerous, is the fact that rather than a limited amount of weighted pull characteristic of supervised bed traction, the vertical traction units subject your spine to the pull exerted by the weight of your entire lower body.

But if you feel that you must try vertical traction, at least temper your enthusiasm with common-sense economics. Holding tightly to any convenient home fixture, such as a door ledge or basement pipe, and suspending yourself by the arms in the fashion of a trapeze artist accomplishes the same result as an expensive vertical traction device.

A second type of unusual traction device frequently advertised as a "miracle cure for back pain" is gravity or moon boots. Several types available that have in common the fact that they necessitate your hanging upside down by your feet, which are held secure by straps or boots. The boots are attached to a frame or rack and, after your feet are secured, the frame is tilted 180 degrees until you are inverted. If this sounds strange, it's probably because it is. And if the technique sounds like an adaptation of the medieval rack, you're right again!

CORSETS AND BRACES

Corsets and braces worn on a bad back are not good for you or your back, particularly when worn for an extended period. But try to tell that to back sufferers with acute and painful muscle spasms and they are not likely to believe you. Why? Because wearing a corset or back brace will probably relieve some of the pain while doing the work of stomach and back muscles for us. This may be a welcome blessing for two or three days, but such devices are likely to compound back problems if are worn over a period of time.

An individual with a painful back who also has weak stomach and back muscles is likely to feel better when the back is at rest. When the back is at rest, these muscles do not have to work and there is generally less pain. Corsets and back braces are designed to hold and support the stomach and back muscles so that they do not have to work as hard to support the spine and, as a result, there is often decreased pain. In addition, weak stomach muscles allow your belly to sag forward, placing extra strain on your already painful back. A corset or brace pulls your stomach in tight and trim. Not only may you feel a bit better, but your friends may ask if you have lost weight! So what's the problem?

The problem is that if the corset or brace is worn over a period of time the already weak stomach and back muscles, which are likely to be contributing to your pain, will quickly become even weaker. The principle is simply that muscles are strengthened by use and exercise and become weaker when they are not used. Corsets and braces restrict back and joint movement and do the work of the abdominal and back muscles. After a time removal of the corset or brace may find you with even more stiffness, soreness, weakness, and hurting than before. This unacceptable situation is remedied only by putting the brace on again. Without it you are worse off than ever as the brace has become a "crutch," and, you may become dependent on the brace to function.

I am reminded of a personal situation that occurred many years ago when I played high school football. During one game I suffered a painful sprained ankle. Within 15 minutes the trainer had strapped my ankle with strong adhesive tape and the previously painful ankle was almost as good as new. I returned to the game with minimal difficulty.

After the game I followed the trainer's advice and kept the ankle securely taped for over a week. Even after removing the strapping, I would stop by the trainer's office each day to have the bad ankle taped before practice and games for the remainder of the season. I recall thinking that the tape made my ankle stronger and I was less likely to suffer another injury. Imagine my surprise when, weeks and months later, my ankle was so weak that it would periodically give out and I would fall on the floor while just walking. It took several months of strengthening exercises before my ankle returned to its original strength.

There are a few instances when corsets or back braces may be essential. People with curved spines (scoliosis) sometimes need a special type of brace designed to correct the curvature, a valuable, conservative device that may help avoid the need for surgery. If a back pain sufferer is unable to strengthen the stomach and back muscles through exercise because of a severe heart condition, hernia, or other medical problem, a corset or brace may need to be permanently worn. However, in the great majority of cases, a corset or brace is a temporary aid at best. You are usually much better off to avoid the brace and get started on an exercise program designed to strengthen the stomach and back muscles (Chapter 10). Avoid laziness! The power to control and relieve your back pain lies with you!

7

DRUG TREATMENT: AN OVERLY MEDICATED SOCIETY?

We're just kinda dopey folks, and we have all these drugs available to us. That's why there's a drug problem, man; there's all these drug stores. It's the biggest thing on the sign—cosmetics, sundries, DRUGS! It's no accident that we're drug oriented, the drug companies got us that way and they'd like to keep us that way. They start you early with the oral habit. Little orange-flavored aspirin for children. "Two in the mouth son." Something wrong with your head? "Two in the mouth, remember that, head–mouth. These are orange. There'll be other colors later on."—George Carlin "FM and AM" Atlantic Records, 1974

Drugs are without question the pain-relief method most commonly employed today. In fact drugs designed for the relief of pain are the most widely used of all pharmacological classes and are of undeniable importance to us. This is not without good reason. They are easy to administer, are relatively inexpensive, and their effects are usually predictable. Drugs are a physician's first line of treatment and they work for many pain patients. For others, unfortunately, drugs serve to multiply the many problems of pain.

Probably the single greatest factor that determines the beneficial or adverse effects of medications in the treatment of back pain is whether the pain is acute or chronic in nature. In Chapter 3 we discussed the major differences between acute and chronic pain. These differences are critical and have major implications with regard to successful treatment and pain relief. First, acute pain describes discomfort from the moment of onset lasting up to six months, while chronic pain lasts six months longer. It is theorized, if not conclusively proved, that different physiologic structures play primary and secondary roles in the transmission of acute and chronic pain impulses in the body. Second, acute pain serves as a warning symptom that something somewhere in the body is amiss and it further serves a protective function in alerting us to take immediate action. Unlike acute pain, chronic pain is not a symptom, but a disease in itself and it has no warning or protective function—it serves no useful purpose whatsoever. Finally, acute pain may be severe and last from moments to several weeks or months, but eventually will subside. Chronic pain may never fully heal, and if treated with medications intended for acute pain, often gets steadily worse.

The problem is this: Although there are numerous and effective analgesic drugs (drugs used to decrease pain) for acute, short-term pain, there are currently no effective painkilling drugs that have been proven safe to take for the many years or lifetime that usually characterizes chronic pain. It is unfortunate that the medicines so effective in the relief of acute pain so often are useless, and even damaging, when used to treat chronic pain. To illustrate this important fact, let us look at two pain victims, Marie and Kenneth.

One year ago, Marie was rushed to the emergency room. While cleaning her home, a water heater had exploded, which sent a ball of fire roaring through the house and leveled several walls and portions of the roof. Marie suffered numerous broken bones from the collapse of the house and serious wounds from flying glass and splinters. In addition, she suffered serious burns over 35 percent of her body. The horrible pain of Marie's initial injuries, as well as the discomfort resulting from three subsequent reconstructive surgeries, was controlled by using powerful narcotic analgesics. Marie now takes no medications for pain and is back caring for her family and enjoying life.

Kenneth was a young man who worked as a carpenter for a local construction company. One day while on the job, he slipped from the roof of a building under construction and fell some ten feet to the ground. Although he landed on his feet and did not sustain any noticeable injuries, the next morning he had trouble getting out of bed because his back was painful and stiff. Kenneth visited his doctor, who diagnosed a back strain and prescribed a mild analgesic and muscle relaxant. The doctor also instructed him to stay in bed for several days of rest. Now, a year later, Kenneth is suffering horrible back pain, is totally disabled from work and most other activities, has been hospitalized on three occasions for diagnostic testing with back strain as the final diagnosis, has been hospitalized once for accidental drug overdose and depression, and each day takes the following medications: Demerol (Winthrop), Talwin, Librium (Roche), Elavil (Merck Sharp & Dohne), Percodan (Endo), Valium (Roche), Motrin (Upjohn), and Soma Compound (Wallace).

Two different patients with two very different treatment outcomes. Marie sustained horribly painful injuries and was treated with some of the most powerful narcotics known, yet one year later was taking no medications for pain and was enjoying an active life. On the other hand, Kenneth experienced a relatively minor injury and was initially treated with mild analgesic medications, yet one year later was essentially an emotional and physical wreck. Why the vastly different results?

The answer is simple: For serious and painful acute disorders, the potential adverse side effects of powerful analgesic drugs are overshadowed by the urgent need to relieve the patient's suffering. In Marie's case there was little hesitation about administering powerful painkilling drugs due to the seriousness of her injuries. Her doctor did not consider it reasonable to worry about her becoming dependent on the narcotic drugs. He realized that although the need for pain relief was urgent, it also was temporary, and there was little risk of causing chemical or psychological dependence in a drug treatment program lasting only a week or two. To minimize this risk further, Marie's doctor carefully monitored her medication intake and quickly and systematically reduced the potency of her medication, until she was taking no drugs at all for pain relief. Marie benefitted from medication during the acute phase of her pain, but her doctor recognized that to continue medications during the long-term phase of pain would be harmful.

Kenneth's case was different. Kenneth was looking for a quick cure and reported to his doctor that he continued to be in pain. His doctor responded by increasing the strength of his medication. When this did not ease the pain, the medications were increased in strength again, but still no results. A different physician was consulted who discontinued one of the medications but added two more, including tranquilizers. In time a third physician was seen and later a surgeon was called in, until it finally became unclear which doctor was prescribing which medication. Kenneth spent most days in a groggy, overmedicated haze. As his body developed a tolerance to each new drug, it took more and more medication to provide relief. In addition, chronic tranquilizer use caused Kenneth to become seriously and clinically depressed. Thus one year after his injury, Kenneth was addicted to several medications, was seriously depressed, and continued to be in pain. Kenneth and his well-intentioned doctors fell into the trap of attempting to treat chronic pain with medications intended for acute pain and he paid a high price for the mistake.

Fortunately more physicians and pain victims are becoming aware that while analgesic drug use in the treatment of acute pain is beneficial, the same medications used to treat chronic pain very often have disastrous effects. In fact there is a growing body of evidence that indicates that many medications traditionally used to relieve pain and suffering can actually prolong and intensify a pain problem. Powerful painkillers can also cause serious toxic side effects when used in high doses for extended periods, and can also result in severe psychological and physical addiction. Furthermore, there is now substantial evidence that powerful analgesic drugs lose their effectiveness for reducing pain after four to six weeks of administration. When this occurs, it soon takes more and more medication to get the same amount of pain relief previously received from only one pill or tablet. Many doctors have looked on in frustration as a patient's chronic pain continues unabated while the patient's drug addiction grows steadily stronger.

Since describing the several hundred different types of drugs that can be used in the treatment of back pain is far beyond the scope of this book, three general classes of frequently used medications will be discussed: narcotic analgesics, nonnarcotic analgesics, and psychotropic drugs. This general overview is intended for informational purposes only. The more informed you are about the advantages and disadvantages of medication for pain control, the better partner you will be with your doctor in deciding on an effective long-term pain management program that works for you. But remember that partners consult on all major decisions and so your doctor should approve and prescribe any medication that you take.

NARCOTIC ANALGESICS

Narcotic drugs are "show stoppers"—the most powerful painkilling and addicting drugs available. Street addicts will rob, steal, and even kill to feed their habit. Back pain victims dependent on narcotics for pain relief will manipulate, lie, doctor-shop, beg, and do practically anything else to fill their need. I echo the opinions of most pain specialists when I state that narcotics have no place in the treatment of chronic benign pain. But all too often some professionals prescribe them and some patients insist on having them.

Most narcotics are opiates; that is, they are derived from opium, a product of the poppy plant, *Papaver somniferum*. The unripe seed capsules are incised and the exudate collected, dried, and powdered. Opium powder contains many alkaloids, such as heroin and methadone, but only morphine, codeine, and papaverine are generally considered to be medically useful. Morphine and codeine are primarily used as analgesics, and papaverine serves as a smooth-muscle relaxant (antispasmodic).

In the past 50 years or so, a number of synthetic derivatives made by modification of the morphine molecule have been manufactured. These derivatives, termed opioids, include Dilaudid (Knoll), Numorphan (Endo), Demerol (Winthrop), and Dolophine (Lilly). These structurally diverse compounds share with morphine the ability to produce analgesia, respiratory depression, gastrointestinal spasm, and physical dependence. None, however, has yet been demonstrated as significantly different from, or superior to, the prototypical narcotic analgesic morphine with respect to their important pharmacology. Morphine thus will be considered as representative of narcotic analgesics.

Morphine and its congeners (synthetically derived compounds) primarily exert their effects on the smooth muscles of the gastrointestinal tract and the central nervous system. Indeed, the use of opium (which contains approximately 10 percent morphine) for relief of diarrhea and dysentery preceded by centuries its use as an analgesic. The effects of morphine on the central nervous system are expressed as a combination of stimulation and depression, and include analgesia, drowsiness, respiratory depression, and depression of the cough reflex.

Morphine-induced analgesia occurs without loss of consciousness and provides only symptomatic relief, without removing or altering the cause of pain. In therapeutic doses there is a tranquilization or mood of calm and drowsiness from which the patient is easily aroused. Subjective effects of morphine and its congeners appear to be dose related. As the dose is increased, drowsiness becomes more pronounced and sleep ensues; the mood of peace and calm will also be accentuated with increased doses. The analgesic effect of narcotic painkillers is also enhanced as the dose is increased so that pain of a more severe nature will be relieved. Unfortunately, as the dose is increased, so too is the incidence of nausea and vomiting and the threat of respiratory depression (decreased or "shallow" breathing, or even the cessation of breathing upon overdose).

Exactly how morphine and its congeners relieve pain is not completely understood at present. Many researchers believe that narcotics produce relief through chemical interactions within central nervous system mechanisms, primarily those of the brain. Opiates interact with receptors, most of which are located in the limbic system of the brain, which in humans is primarily associated with the arousal of emotions. Rather than altering the peripheral chemical interaction or sensations that are responsible for sending pain messages to the brain, it is believed that narcotics work by changing the affective component of the pain experience. For example, after administration of a narcotic analgesic, you may report that your back pain continues but is no longer discomforting, or that the pain can be tolerated much easier and with calm or indifference. This explains the calm, mellow, or what is frequently referred to as the "don't give a damn" attitude of patients receiving narcotic medications.

One of the more serious drawbacks of narcotic analgesic use is the threat of tolerance and physical dependence. Tolerance is defined as a decreased responsiveness to any drug as the result of prior administrations of the drug. More simply stated, after taking a narcotic drug for a period of time, the human body adapts and the drug loses some of its effectiveness. Consequently, increasingly larger doses must be administered to produce a level of pain relief equivalent to that of the initial administration. Many pain victims and physicians have innocently fallen victim of the "tolerance trap" whereby pain relief is sought through steadily increasing doses of narcotic drugs until dependency occurs.

Physical dependence refers to an abnormal physiological state produced by repeated administration of a drug, which then makes necessary the continued use of the drug to prevent the appearance of a withdrawal or abstinence syndrome. This threat is particularly meaningful to the chronic pain patient who suffers months or years of discomfort and frequently searches for stronger and stronger drugs to kill the pain. A primary goal of many chronic pain programs is to withdraw the pain sufferer gradually from a physical dependence on narcotic analgesic drugs. A sad situation exists when an individual with a problem of chronic back pain seeks relief with medications, only to compound the situation by developing a drug dependency. When this occurs, as it does quite frequently, the victim becomes saddled with two problems—chronic back pain and drug dependency.

Codeine, like morphine and aspirin, is a naturally occurring substance and is often used to treat moderate to severe pain. Also like morphine and other opiates, codeine can cause adverse side effects, including depressed breathing, nausea and vomiting, dizziness, constipation, drowsiness, and sedation. For this reason patients taking codeine or other powerful medications should be very careful when performing activities that require alertness or fast reaction time, such as driving an automobile. In addition, care should be exercised to ensure that other drugs that cause drowsiness are not taken with codeine since the additive effect is potentially very dangerous. Codeine may not be as habit forming as morphine, but prolonged use can lead to increased tolerance and ultimately to addiction.

Demerol (meperidine, Winthrop) is a wholly synthetic analgesic and sedative supposedly free of many of morphine's undesirable side effects. Demerol does not significantly differ from morphine in its important pharmacology. In therapeutic doses it produces pain relief, sedation, and respiratory depression, as well as the other central nervous system actions mentioned as common to other narcotic analgesics. With regard to its supposed lack of undesirable properties, it should be noted that Demerol is the narcotic most commonly abused by health professionals in treating back pain, who still mistakenly believe that it has a lower threat of causing physical dependence and is easier to stop using than morphine. In fact Demerol abuse and dependence have been widely documented since the drug was first introduced, and it is now recognized that Demerol differs little from morphine with respect to its potential for abuse and dependence. Demerol is perhaps the most frequently abused medication among chronic back pain victims treated at our centers.

Darvon (propoxyphene, Lilly) is also a wholly synthetic agent that is often used with patients who cannot tolerate codeine. At present Darvon is legally classified as a "nonnarcotic" and is usually prescribed as an analgesic for mild to moderate pain. Its legal status notwithstanding, Darvon is classified under narcotic analgesics in this chapter because it is subject to abuse. Physical dependence can also develop during high-dose chronic use. There is no great difference between the dependence liabilities of codeine and Darvon.

Despite the adverse side effects described, narcotic medications are relatively safe drugs when prescribed for *short-term* use by a knowledgable physician and remain the standard drugs of choice in the treatment of many acute and severe pain states such as postoperative pain, multiple trauma, and the acute pain of heart attacks. However, narcotic drugs have few, if any, appropriate uses in the treatment of chronic benign back pain. As doctors become increasingly aware of the contraindications of narcotic use in intractable pain, many experts in the field of pain management expect the use and abuse of habit-forming drugs in the treatment of chronic pain states to decrease substantially.

When your back hurts so badly that you would do practically anything for relief, be particularly careful that the "anything" does not include taking narcotic drugs. The temptation will be great since narcotics are powerful enough to stop the pain and also provide you with a euphoric "high" that is appealing to many pain victims tired of fighting the daily frustration and drain of chronic pain. But if you are a victim of chronic back pain, taking narcotic drugs for pain relief is like pouring gasoline on a burning fire.

Detoxification

Are you physically or psychologically dependent on medications? Take a moment to read the following questions and give them some serious and honest thought before answering.

1. Do you take medications for pain five or more days per week?
2. Do you feel calmer, more relaxed, and happier when you take medications?
3. Do you take medications before plans to be around groups, such as family and friends?
4. Can you sleep without taking medications before going to bed?
5. Do you get up during the night to take medications?
6. If you do not take your medication as prescribed, do you feel nervous, tense, or anxious?
7. How would you react if someone suddenly took all of your medication away from you?

If you believe you may be dependent on medications, don't panic! Over 40 percent of the patients treated in our program have inadvertently become dependent on one or more medications. In an effort to stop hurting, these individuals have sometimes spent months and years experimenting with a variety of doctors and therapies, and nothing works. During their long and fruitless search for a solution, many have become either physically or psychologically dependent on drugs.

Physical dependency on medication is a biochemical and physiological problem; your body craves medications and requires that you take them. The human body becomes accustomed to drugs and, over time, needs certain addicting drugs as it needs air and water. Because physical dependency causes certain chemical changes, the body will experience withdrawal symptoms without the substance on which it has come to depend. These symptoms can include shakes, sweats, cramps, and convulsions. Long-term use of addicting drugs can lead to marked and drastic changes in personality and, in some cases, can produce permanent residual brain damage.

Psychological dependency on medications is an emotional problem that can have physical symptoms as a result. Drugs that reduce physical suffering, and particularly those medications that also reduce anxiety, assist in sleep, and have a calming, pleasant effect, have a strong potential for abuse. When you hurt less and feel more relaxed and tranquil, your body and brain are both happy. If simply swallowing a small pill was responsible for the escape from turmoil, agitation, frustration, and pain, there is a strong tendency to swallow another, and then another. In time your entire body comes to expect this more pleasant state and you begin to anticipate situations that may upset the chemical tranquility. For example, you have an important appointment in the morning so you need a good night's sleep. Or your family is coming over for Sunday lunch and that always makes you a bit anxious. Maybe the children will be out of school on Saturday and you know they will get on your nerves. Or you have an appointment to discuss your taxes with an accountant and that is always frustrating.

Once you begin to anticipate situations that may cause increased tension, frustration, anxiety, and pain, you may then begin to prepare yourself for these situations by taking more medication than usual. You may even try to justify your behavior by playing mind games: "Taking a little more medication will keep me from hurting so badly and will help keep me relaxed; my family will have more fun if I'm not on edge." Before long you have a psychological dependency and the thought of running out of your drugs, or even leaving them at home for several hours while going shopping ("What if I need them?"), creates a psychological panic reaction with subsequent physical symptoms of increased pain, anxiety, tension, and body aches. Life soon revolves around the anticipation of potential mind or body upset and preparation for it by swallowing chemical "protection."

In our programs we use "pain cocktails" to withdraw victims from addicting medications. There are five different cocktails, A, B, C, D, and E. The cocktails are identical in volume, appearance, taste, and color so that they cannot be distinguished from one another. Cocktail A is the most potent and contains powerful narcotic ingredients. Cocktail B is also quite strong, but not as potent as cocktail A. Cocktails C and D have decreased amounts of active ingredients while cocktail E has no medication in it (only liquid vitamins and taste-masking elixir).

At our centers we start patients dependent on medication on cocktail A or B and then gradually work them down to cocktail E. The entire withdrawal process takes approximately 20 days and all withdrawal symptoms are avoided. The majority of pain victims, initially terrified by anticipated severe pain without strong analgesic medications, are pleasantly surprised to discover that they have much less pain on no medication than they suffered while on powerful, addicting drugs.

It should be clearly understood that while the intent of this book is to help yourself better manage low back pain, it is definitely not recommended that you attempt to withdraw yourself from medications for pain without first consulting your physician. The symptoms of drug withdrawal can be quite serious and you may require hospitalization in order to be medically monitored during withdrawal. Discuss a drug withdrawal plan with your physician and follow his or her advice. It is almost certain that with chronic noncancerous low back pain, drug elimination will do far more than any medication toward allowing you to experience less pain and to feel more alert, confident, and better able to cope with your disorder.

NONNARCOTIC ANALGESICS

Drugs classified as nonnarcotic analgesics constitute a large and varied group of compounds far too extensive to address adequately within the limitations of this chapter. Therefore, only selected drugs (those that are widely used and those with potentially unique applications in low back pain problems) will be discussed. For our purposes we can divide these medications into two broad categories: proprietary (or over-the-counter) drugs and prescription medications.

Proprietary Drugs

Proprietary analgesics are also referred to as over-the-counter drugs since they can be purchased without a prescription. But do not make the mistake of believing that just because the medications are readily available, they are worthless for reducing pain or are harmless and can be taken at will. Many proprietary drugs are surprisingly effective in controlling discomfort but can also be abused and have serious harmful side effects. In general you should not self-medicate without the advice of a physician if you:

1. Have asthma or other allergic diseases.
2. Have stomach ulcers.
3. Have had past allergic reactions to aspirin or other pain medications.
4. Take medications that affect blood clotting.
5. Have a history of gout, arthritis, or diabetes.

There conditions represent instances where medications may have adverse effects on underlying disorders. In addition, the presence of any of these factors should strongly encourage you to consult your physician.

Aspirin

Aspirin (acetylsalicylic acid) is a highly effective and important member of those analgesics classified as nonnarcotics and, moreover, is the single most widely used drug in the world, narcotic or nonnarcotic. In addition to its use as a pain reliever, aspirin has antipyretic (reduces fever) and anti-inflammation (reduces noninfectious redness and swelling) properties. Because aspirin is a nonprescription drug and easily accessible, it is not always credited with the analgesic efficacy it possesses. When compared with other analgesics, aspirin is effective, useful, and inexpensive, and has a relatively low incidence of adverse side effects.

Aspirin and other nonnarcotic analgesics appear to reduce pain by interfering with the biochemistry of pain formation at peripheral nerve sites in the body. Unlike narcotic analgesics, aspirin does not alter the response to pain in the central nervous system, and therefore it has a lower analgesic effect. For example, 650 mg (milligrams) of aspirin is generally thought to produce as much pain relief as 60 mg of codeine. Doses of aspirin exceeding 650 mg, however, do not increase peak analgesia (although the duration of the effect may be prolonged), whereas increased doses of codeine will provide greater relief from pain. Aspirin, it seems, has a "ceiling effect" at around 600 mg, and doses beyond that amount do little to increase its effectiveness. Aspirin may have some slight effects on central nervous system activity, but compared with the effects of morphine and other narcotic analgesics, they are negligible.

Although aspirin is relatively safe, does not cause physical dependence, and is readily available, it can produce side effects, such as heartburn, nausea, gastric (stomach) irritation, and possibly gastric bleeding. Aspirin also reduces the tendency of blood to clot, thereby prolonging bleeding time. Significant overmedication can cause aspirin toxicity, which can be fatal. The symptoms of extreme aspirin poisoning include hypothermia (loss of body heat), cardiac arrhythmia (irregular heartbeat), shallow breathing, coma, and death. When properly treated, however, most cases of aspirin poisoning are not life-threatening. Ringing in the ears or dizziness may signal approaching toxicity; if you experience either condition, contact your physician.

Aspirin tablets should be taken with eight ounces of water after meals, or if appropriate, with an antacid. All aspirin should be kept in a tightly closed bottle in a cool dry place and out of reach of children. The bathroom is not a good place to store aspirin because of dampness. Throw away any aspirin that smells like vinegar.

There are numerous proprietary analgesic medications available whose primary active chemical ingredient is aspirin.

Plain aspirin tablets differ primarily in price as they are usually similarly manufactured. However, there are a some products that are not as well manufactured as others and can be either too hard or too soft. Tightly compressed tablets do not dissolve readily, whereas loose, crumbled tablets can contain degraded drugs. These products often have a vinegary odor and should not be taken since they have pharmaceutical differences that can be clinically important.

Buffered aspirin theoretically offers some advantage as an analgesic because of the stomach irritation associated with unbuffered aspirin. This product is usually more expensive than plain aspirin.

Buffered aspirin solutions (usually liquid) can give rapid and effective relief, although they generally increase urinary excretion of salicylate. The large sodium content and decrease in salicylate blood levels make these products unsuitable for long-term administration, but very effective for occasional treatment of low back pain.

Enteric-coated aspirin are coated with a substance that does not dissolve until it reaches the intestine, where the drug is then released. Since it takes longer to produce pain relief, this type of medication is not generally used for the treatment of acute back pain, though it is most appropriate for patients with a history of ulcers or severe gastric distress.

Some *aspirin combinations* contain phenacitin and/or caffeine and may be less effective than other available preparations. In addition, aspirin combinations are thought to produce more adverse side effects and usually are not considered most appropriate for treatment of chronic back pain.

Extra-strength pain relievers are available in two general types. The first type contains more than one analgesic in a single product, and the total ingredient of aspirin usually exceeds 325 mg. The second type usually contains more than 325 mg of the same drug. Often one "extra-strength" preparation is nearly equal to two capsules or tablets of regular strength; therefore, it is often implied that "extra-strength" drugs are more effective, although results vary. The primary advantage of this type of medication may be that you swallow fewer capsules or tablets.

Acetaminophen (Datril, Tylenol, Liquiprin, and Others)*

Acetaminophen is approximately equal in analgesic strength to aspirin and has a mode of action in the body that is also similar to aspirin. Acetaminophen has enjoyed a surge of popularity in recent years as an effective analgesic that does not cause the gastric irritation and bleeding that can result from aspirin intake.

Acetaminophen is both an analgesic and antipyretic. The analgesic effect is achieved with one (325 mg) or two tablets. Taking

*Datril (Bristol-Myers), Tylenol (McNeil Consumer Products), Liquiprin (Morcliff Thayer)

more tablets is useless and perhaps dangerous, depending on the quantity and the individual. In excessive doses acetaminophen can cause fatal liver damage (excessive in this case can be as few as 30 tablets taken in a relatively short period of time). As mentioned, aspirin can also be fatally abused, but it is a much slower-acting analgesic. Overdose of aspirin follows a progressive pattern into coma and shock. For occasional relief of backache, acetaminophen can be an effective medication.

If you take acetaminophen for pain relief, be careful not to exceed the specific dosage and dosing intervals. Ten to 60 minutes is usually required for this drug to be effective and the effects will normally last from six to eight hours. You should not take acetaminophen regularly for more than ten days without consulting your physician.

Prescription Drugs

Anti-inflammatory Medication (Motrin, Dolobid, Indocin, and others)*

These medications were initially designed for reducing the tissue swelling that occurs with certain forms of arthritis. As so frequently happens with new types of manufactured drugs, a secondary advantage soon became known. In the case of anti-inflammatory drugs, not only do they reduce tissue swelling, but they seem to reduce pain as well. A large number of well-known medications routinely used to treat various medical disorders were originally manufactured and marketed for other disorders.

Anti-inflammatory medications are sometimes effective in reducing the discomfort of selected back disorders. Unfortunately these drugs cause rather severe nausea and vomiting in many people who try them. Heartburn and allergic reactions are also possible, though less frequent, side effects. Dizziness, blurring of vision, and easy bruising should be reported to your doctor.

Muscle Relaxants (Robaxin, Soma, Parafon Forte, and Others)*

When you are in pain, particularly with low back pain, the mus-

---

*Motrin (Upjohn), Dolobid (Merck Sharp & Dohne), Indocin (Merck Sharp & Dohne)
*Robaxin (Robins), Soma (Wallace), Parafon Forte (McNeil)

cles throughout your body have a tendency to tighten and contract. This is an involuntary response that many scientists believe is an evolutional carryover trait from cave people who generally experienced pain only when physically attacked. Since the cave dweller was forced either to fight or flee when attacked and injured, his or her muscles involuntarily contracted in preparation for action. It seems that we today continue to demonstrate much of our early heritage. If you don't believe it, watch carefully the next time someone drops a heavy object on a toe. You may notice that the muscles immediately tighten and contract, which prepares the victim for the action of holding one foot while wildly hopping around (fleeing?) on the other. Even with our twentieth century sophistication, there are occasional reminders that we are all products of infinite years of reflex heredity.

When you suffer back pain, the paraspinal muscles that run along both sides of the spinal column seem particularly prone to tightening and contracting. As we have previously discussed, muscles that contract and stay tight for periods of time cause pain. This can be easily demonstrated by tightening your hand into a fist and holding the muscle tension until your hand begins to hurt. As you can imagine, the problems of an already painful back are compounded by involuntary muscular contraction and the result is a great deal of discomfort.

Muscle relaxant medications are intended to do just what their name implies—relax muscles. Unfortunately muscle relaxants relax not only the muscles in the back, but muscles all over the body, and therein lies one of the problems with these drugs. Add frequent nausea and dizziness to the sleepy, weak, tired, confused, and lithargic feelings produced by overall body chemical relaxation, and it is seen that muscle relaxant drugs seldom provide an adequate solution to the problems of back pain.

PSYCHOTROPIC MEDICATIONS

An important third category of drugs is termed psychotropic and has been recognized only recently as often effective in the treatment of chronic pain states. Psychotropic drugs can be defined as agents that affect our mood, behavior, or experience and are most commonly employed in psychiatric practice. In the past few years, however, psychotropic drugs (hypnotics, sedatives, stimulants, antianxiety drugs, and antidepressants) have found a place in the treatment of chronic pain. For our purposes we will briefly discuss two major subcategories of psychotropic medications frequently used in the treatment of back pain—antianxiety and antidepressant drugs.

Antianxiety Medications (Valium, Librium, Serax, Tranxene, and Others)*

One of the many variables that must be taken into account when a physician prescribes a medication for pain, including back pain, is to what extent the patient's anxiety may be causing or intensifying the pain. Again we are reminded of the pain–tension cycle described throughout this text and the very important roles that stress, tension, and anxiety play in back discomfort. These considerations form part of the foundation of this book, as well as much of the treatment for chronic back pain offered in our pain therapy programs.

Tranquilizers are manufactured and prescribed to reduce anxiety, which sounds good and simple enough. And there are volumes of research to indicate that, in fact, they do just what they are intended to do. But we seldom get something for nothing and, in the case of medications, few things are that simple and straightforward. So what price will you pay to tranquilize your frayed nerves chemically?

One of the problems with certain tranquilizers, such as Valium; is the effect that these drugs have on your body chemistry and the subsequent effect on your pain. When taken over a period of time, many tranquilizers are thought to alter the effects of serotonin (one of the body's natural chemicals) in the brain. Since serotonin is involved in sleep, pain tolerance, and our emotional stability, prolonged tranquilizer use is thought to interfere with our natural ability to sleep and tolerate pain. Prolonged intake can also cause depression. In addition, some tranquilizers are habit forming. In the past few years, several books and movies have been released that describe the agony of tranquilizer addiction. At our centers we frequently see individuals whose back pain resolves but who are left with a residue of drug dependency.

*Valium (Roche), Librium (Roche), Serax (Wyeth), Tranxene (Abbott)

Are tranquilizers the answer to your back pain problem? I hope you agree that the answer is no!

Antidepressant Medications (Elavil, Sinequan, Tofranil, and Others)*

The use of antidepressant medications for chronic back pain is a new, but promising, application of these drugs. There are basically three types of antidepressant medication available: tricyclic antidepressants, monomine oxidase inhibitors, and psychostimulants. Only tricyclic drugs are employed in the treatment of chronic pain.

Chronic pain and depression have a complex but undeniable association with each other. But which comes first, the pain or the depression? Certainly it is not difficult to understand how the daily torture of living with a constantly aching back can gradually wear a victim down to a state of helplessness, despair, and depression. The same can be said for dealing with any chronic problem. But there is also a substantial amount of recent research to suggest that depressed individuals suffer more injuries and pain than people who are not depressed. On a less scientific basis, this suggestion is evidenced by the fact that most individuals admitted to psychiatric hospitals for primary depression also have complaints of chronic pain that greatly exceed the pain complaints of the general population. Thus does chronic pain cause depression or do depressed individuals develop chronic pain?

The answer, I think, is neither and both. First, there is no direct, foolproof causal relationship between chronic back pain and depression. I suppose that it is possible that a victim could suffer chronic back pain and not become depressed, although we seldom see this exceptional individual in any of our programs. It is also possible, and even probable, that there are clinically depressed individuals with no complaints of pain. As a result there is no direct causal relationship between chronic pain and depression or depression and pain that holds true for every individual.

On the other hand, we cannot simply ignore the obvious relationship between chronic pain and depression that exists in a great number of victims. As mentioned, it is easy to understand how prolonged pain can ultimately lead to depression. We also cannot

*Elavil (Merck Sharp & Dohne), Sinequan (Roerig), Tofranil (Geigy)

ignore the research evidence that tells us that more individuals suffering depression ultimately suffer painful back injuries and pain than nondepressed individuals. Perhaps the answer is that some persons suffer depression as a result of chronic pain, while others suffer recognized or unrecognized depression that heralds the onset of injury or pain. If this is true, perhaps the common link between our two types of victims is one of the brain's natural biochemicals called *serotonin*.

Serotonin is a natural chemical that is known to play a major role in both depression and pain (as well as sleep). Research has suggested that when there is a reduction of serotonin in the brain, most individuals will suffer sleep problems and either depression, increased pain, or both. We do not fully understand why serotonin is sometimes reduced, but we do know that drugs such as Valium and certain drugs taken for high blood pressure can alter the supply of serotonin in the brain. This is why I pointed out earlier that the majority of doctors who specialize in the treatment of pain are strongly opposed to the use of Valium and related drugs to control the anxiety and muscle spasms associated with chronic pain. The use of such drugs decreases the supply of serotonin in the brain and may result in increased pain, serious depression, and sleep disturbance.

But if reducing the supply of serotonin causes depression and increased pain, should not drugs that increase the supply of serotonin relieve depression, decrease pain, and improve sleep? The answer is yes, and the name given to one such category of drugs is tricyclic antidepressants. Particularly when taken before retiring, many of these drugs can immediately improve sleep and provide mild relaxation and, after two or three weeks of administration, can often reduce depression and chronic pain. You may initially experience some mild dryness of the mouth and constipation, but this normally goes away in a week or so. When taken as properly prescribed, antidepressant medication is generally a safe, nonaddicting, and effective aid to control chronic back pain. When used in combination with the overall back care program outlined in this book, antidepressant medication is thought by many to represent the safest and most effective drug available for chronic back discomfort. As with many drugs, it should be noted that antidepressant medication is potentially lethal if taken in excess.

What is our cost for chemical pain control through the use of narcotic, anti-inflammatory, muscle relaxant, and tranquilizing drugs? Let us add up the bill: natural sleep interference, reduced natural ability to tolerate pain, mental confusion, psychological depression, nausea, lack of energy, potential drug addiction. Is the cost too great? You be the judge. But before you decide, keep in mind that this book is filled with nonsurgical, nonmedication techniques that have been proven effective in helping you to control pain, anxiety, and depression, as well as to increase your activities and live a more normal and productive life. And the only cost is the time and effort required to learn and practice the techniques described. You decide.

8

THE RARE NEED FOR SURGERY

To many sufferers from back pain, the word surgery is synonymous with relief. They don't care to waste time on "lesser" treatments when the "magic knife" will cure the problem. They also have little interest in seeing any rehabilitation or primary care doctors. These individuals want a surgeon who, in their eyes, is the only "real doctor" capable of effectively managing as serious a case as their pain problem—and not only a surgeon, but the type of surgeon we see on television who is called in on a case when all other nonsurgeon doctors are baffled and perplexed. This "savior" usually would be young, handsome, and aggressive. Ideally, he would spend about two minutes examining you before shouting an order for emergency surgery, scold the other doctors and nurses for their incompetence, and finally rest a gentle hand on your shoulder and reassure you that he is going to eliminate your pain and suffering. He might also guarantee to save your life, remove a few corns and callouses from your feet, run a complete check on your back and internal organs to ensure proper functioning, and perhaps throw in a face-lift at no extra cost. Not only will you feel better, but you will look better and you will have him to thank for your new lease on life.

Are there surgeons who fit this description? There may well be a few scattered about. Are there back pain victims who really want surgery and even the surgeon described? In my opinion the answer is an unequivocable yes!

The belief that back surgery is a guaranteed cure-all for pain, that the degree of pain intensity dictates the decision to operate, or that surgery is a means of "getting it all over with quickly" and avoiding the need for further back care, has no basis in reality. Surgery is a treatment technique for *specific* back problems and should not be considered the treatment of last resort if all other nonsurgical treatments fail. The simple fact is that surgery can help only a fraction of all back pain victims and, except for a few diagnosed disorders, should be avoided if possible.

Doctors' (as well as most surgeons') reluctance to operate on one's back is based on sound principles of anatomy, physiology, and psychology, and on simple fact. If you believe that surgery is the only treatment that will cure your back problem, take a few minutes to review what I call the "five facts of back surgery." They are *not* presented in an attempt to convince you to refuse needed surgery, but as information. Many health-care professionals believe that health care is most successful when the doctor and patient work together. To be an active participant in decisions affecting your health, you must know the facts.

1. The great majority of back problems can be more effectively managed with many of the treatment techniques described in this book than with surgery. In addition, these techniques do not expose the patient to the potential risks of surgery.
2. Surgery is unlikely to cure your back pain in the sense that a surgical appendectomy can cure appendicitis pain. Most patients who undergo back surgery find that they still have some pain following even successful surgery. For example, suppose you suffer a herniated disk that presses on a nerve and causes low back pain and discomfort radiating down the leg. Surgery may eliminate the leg pain, but you may continue to suffer pain in the lower back.
3. Back surgery will seldom give you a "normal" back. No matter what is creating your back discomfort, you are almost certain to come out of surgery with some part of your spine removed or some once-movable joint permanently immobilized. In fact, the anatomical and physiological changes that are an unavoidable part of surgery may cause or contribute to new back pain and future problems.
4. Successful back surgery may depend as much, or more, on the doctor's diagnostic capability than on surgical expertise. We have learned that pain is a psychophysiological phenomenon with both psychological and psychophysiological components (Chapters 3 and 4). The psychological variables that influence the cause and perception of pain are totally normal reactions to which we all are subject, usually at the unconscious level. Let me again emphasize that I am not discussing pain that is "all in the head" or "faked." The psychophysiological nature of chronic pain is a normal process of which most victims are not aware. Since even the most highly skilled surgeon cannot "cut out" the psychological component of pain and suffering, all factors influencing back pain must be diagnosed accurately prior to making the decision to operate. For example, scientific research has well documented the fact that back surgery on patients receiving compensation for pain and injury is only about half as successful as back surgery performed on noncompensated pain victims.

5. Surgery is no substitute for a lifelong program of sensible back care. This does not mean that I am totally against back surgery. In carefully selected individuals who suffer a very limited number of painful disorders, back surgery can produce dramatic and effective results. However, I am against the popular notion that back surgery will inevitably end in either triumph or tragedy. In the vast majority of cases, the outcome will be somewhere between these two extremes. If you are a candidate for back surgery, it is important that you consider surgery not as "magic" but simply as the first step in the management of your back. With this realization, and the determination to follow through with the therapeutic plan, you are less likely to be disappointed by the results of an operation.

For those few patients who will benefit from back surgery, the significant details of the technique should be discussed. There are basically two types of surgery for back disorders: decompression and stabilization.

Decompression surgery may be performed on patients with a disk pressing against a nerve or those who suffer back pain as the result of a nerve being impinged by bone. Usually a bulging disk is responsible for pressure on a nerve root (where the nerve leaves the spine), or less commonly a piece of disk may break loose and press against a nerve. In a few cases, the nerve impingement results not from disc fragments, but from a bony prominence that pushes on a nerve or partially closes the canal in which a spinal nerve passes. We will briefly discuss two types of decompression surgery, *diskectomy* and *laminectomy*.

Stabilization surgery is performed to eliminate spinal weakness or motion that may result in back pain. Stabilization surgery is usually termed spinal fusion.

DISKECTOMY

Surgery to relieve disk pressure involves removal of part of the disk, a technique termed discectomy. If you are scheduled for a diskectomy, this is what you can expect.

You will usually be asked to check into the hospital a day or so before surgery. If you have not previously undergone a myelogram (Chapter 5), perhaps one will be scheduled prior to surgery. There will be the usual blood and urine laboratory tests and a routine physical examination by your surgeon or another physician the day prior to surgery. On the evening before surgery, you will be given medication to help you sleep and informed that you are not to eat or drink after midnight. This restriction prevents possible complications with anesthesia.

On the morning of surgery, you will be given an injection to help you relax before being taken to the operating room. In the operating room, you may be vaguely aware of where you are and your environment but you will be quite relaxed and calm. In time an anesthesiologist or nurse anethetist will administer general anesthesia and you will "go to sleep." You will be placed on your stomach so that you may breathe easily and so that your back is accessible to the surgeon.

The surgeon will begin the operation by making a two- or three-inch incision over the area of your troublesome disk, and then continue through, around, over, and under layers of muscle, bone, and ligaments. After removing a small portion of the roof of the spinal canal, the nerve root and disk are visible. The surgeon surveys the small area for loose pieces of disk and removes them. Next the disk is explored, much like a blowout in a tire, from which some of the contents may have escaped. A special instrument is used to enlarge the hole and clean out any remaining contents of the damaged disk. It is usually impossible to remove all of the contents, but as much as possible is taken out.

The surgical closing is relatively simple. First the nerve root and muscles, which have been temporarily pushed aside, are replaced in their proper position and the muscles are sutured. Next the incision is brought together and stitched. The entire procedure generally takes from 60 to 90 minutes.

You are then taken to the recovery room, where you gradually regain consciousness. You may experience some nausea and vomiting from the anesthesia but this can be controlled with medication. When you are fairly alert and medically stable, you will be taken back to your room and asked to lie on your back. You may sleep for several hours under the careful watch of the nurses.

Your back will be quite painful for several days following surgery. This discomfort is primarily from back muscles that are unavoidably bruised during the operation. The pain can be controlled with medication. In a day or so, you should be feeling much improved since diskectomy is the least disruptive to your system of any type of major back surgery.

Many patients are surprised that they are encouraged to walk to the restroom on the evening of surgery. The day following surgery is an active time and you will be encouraged to stand most of the day, up and walking. You will probably be discharged from the hospital in four to seven days with instructions to get plenty of rest but also to walk each day. Depending on what you do for a living, you may be back at work in three to six weeks.

LAMINECTOMY

Another variation of decompression surgery occurs when bone, rather than a protruding disk, presses against a sensitive spinal nerve. The spinal canal may have "overgrown" due to aging, and be cramping the nerves. Perhaps a disk has narrowed and allowed the vertebrae above and below the disk to settle together too closely and press on a nerve. Perhaps a developed bony spur is the culprit.

In these various disorders, the decompression surgical technique is essentially the same as that described for a herniated disk. The procedure, termed laminectomy, involves surgically removing the lamina (the roof of the spinal canal). This technique differs from the discectomy in that the surgeon removes an offending section of bone or enlarges an exit canal, depending upon what is exerting pressure on the nerve, but the disk is usually left intact.

A laminectomy usually takes 60–90 minutes to complete and you may be hospitalized for five to ten days. If a great amount of bone was removed, you may be instructed to wear a back brace or corset for several weeks until your back regains its strength. Returning to your job, again depends on the type of work performed, but it can usually be resumed within a couple of months.

SPINAL FUSION

Spinal fusion is a surgical procedure in which two separate bones in the back are "fused" or united to prevent motion at the joint between them. Spinal fusions are performed less frequently than diskectomies or laminectomies. Two major side effects of spinal fusion that should be fully realized and considered prior to the surgery are that the operation will seldom relieve all of your back pain and your back will lose a portion of its flexibility after two or more vertebrae are "welded" together.

If you are a candidate for spinal fusion, this is what you can expect. The preliminary admission, laboratory work, physical examination, and anesthesia are the same as for diskectomy. For a variety of reasons, spinal fusion may occasionally be performed from the front of the body, particularly when vertebrae in the neck are to be fused. However, most fusions for lower back problems are performed from the back. The incision is similar to that used in diskectomy and laminectomy, except larger.

The surgeon will next cut through or push aside muscles and ligaments until the spinal vertebrae are exposed. The vertebrae will then be scuffed and abraded with an instrument similar to a carpenter's chisel. This deliberate damage activates the same inherent tendency of bone that allows a fractured arm or broken leg to heal and assists in the fusion process.

Since sections of bone must be used to bridge the vertebrae together and allow fusion, and since your own bone runs the least chance of being rejected by your body, a bone donor site must be located. A favorite is the iliac crest or hip bone. An incision is made and the surgeon carves ten to 15 small strips of bone, each about the size of a match stick. The small bone strips are then strategically placed to attach to the vertebrae being fused. The bone strips will die; their purpose is to act as a lattice or framework over and through which bone cells in the two vertebrae can grow. When the bone graft is complete, the bones become one.

Recovery from spinal fusion is much slower than from diskectomy and laminectomy. The bone growth process is much like that in the healing of a fracture; and as with fracture healing, the growth may be slow. You will probably be hospitalized for about two weeks and ordered home to rest for an additional two to three months. In some cases it takes as long as six months before a solid fusion is achieved. Also, as with some fractures, bones sometimes do not fuse. When this infrequent problem does occur, a new fusion operation must be performed.

During the postsurgical phase, your back must be treated with a degree of special care. Years ago doctors would put spinal fusion patients in a body cast of plaster to prevent movement until the fusion was solid. We now know that the recently fused back does not have to be treated like a delicate china antique, but the success of fusion does depend on your ability to keep the newly fused joints reasonably undisturbed. You will be required to wear a back brace and cautioned to move about easily and to avoid any stress on the spine.

A few final words about spinal fusion. First, spinal fusion is major surgery involving a lengthy recovery. More than twice as many complications occur with spinal fusion as with diskectomy and there is a 20 percent chance that the bones will not fuse. Since the recommendation of fusion is often a judgment call on the doctor's part, a second opinion is certainly your prerogative and an excellent idea. Second, spinal fusion does *not* make your back stronger, but more rigid. You will lose some of the flexibility of the spine following surgery and should be prepared to anticipate in a lifetime back care program. Third, spinal fusion places an increased strain on the spinal structures above and below the fusion. This increased strain can cause problems in the future. Finally, spinal fusion is unlikely to eliminate your back pain completely or to spell the end of your troublesome back. The advantages and disadvantages of surgery should be considered carefully before deciding to undergo spinal fusion.

CHEMONUCLEOLYSIS

One of the newst techniques in the war against back pain is not actually a surgical procedure although surgeons perform the great majority of treatments. Chemonucleolysis is technically termed a "closed surgical procedure" and has been practiced for years in Canada, Europe, and the Soviet Union, but was only recently approved by the Federal Drug Administration (FDA) for use in the United States. There is a great deal of debate over the usefulness and safety of this technique and the controversy is far from settled.

Chemonucleolysis essentially means destroying the inner nucleus of a spinal disk (nucleus pulposus) by injecting into the disk a chemical called chymopapain which is marketed under the trade name of Chymodiactin. Chymopapain is a chemical derived from the leaves of the papaya plant. The enzymes' ability to digest cartilage has been known for centuries; in fact, for years Polynesians have wrapped meat in papaya leaves to make it more tender.

Intradiscal therapy, as the technique of injecting chymopapain is sometimes called, is approved by the FDA only for treatment of herniated disks of the lumbar spine. In a series of recent one-day workshops at which over 7000 physicians were instructed in the technique of intradiskal therapy, the workshop sponsors (American Academy of Orthopaedic Surgeons and American Association of Neurological Surgeons) listed three aspects for selection of candidates for chymopapain injections. The first is an adequate trial of conservative management, defined as complete bed rest, analgesic medications, and physical therapy for two to four weeks. Those who continue with unremitting pain and are unable to perform everyday activities or return to work are candidates for further therapy.

The second component should be definite radiating pain or numbness down the leg following the anatomical distribution of a nerve. There should also be a straight leg raise test that is positive for pain on the involved side or depression of a deep tendon reflex (Chapter 5).

The third criterion is that an abnormal myelogram should confirm disk herniation at the appropriate level, although the use of a CT scan or electromyography (EMG) is also permitted. The workshop syllabus further suggests that chymopapain injection be considered only in cases of lumbar disk herniation with associated impingement on a nerve root. The technique is not recommended in the treatment of spondylosis on spinal stenosis (Chapter 4), or when bony spurs are responsible for the nerve entrapment.

As previously mentioned, there remains a great deal of controversy regarding the effectiveness of chemonucleolysis. Many authorities simply do not believe that the injection of chymopapain has the therapeutic effect that proponents report and also question the long-term effects of what some describe as 20 or more years of disk aging that takes place within minutes of intradiskal therapy. Scientific research has also failed to give us unequivocable results since many studies report the technique as highly effective while others report intradiskal therapy as no more effective than placebo treatment. Certainly the fact that, in light of poor results from controlled investigations in 1975, one drug manufacturer withdrew its new drug application pending before the FDA, even though the company had a vested economic interest in seeing chymopapain approved, does little to instill our confidence in the drug. The FDA approved chymopapain for use in the United States in the early 1980s.

A chymopapain injection has side effects, the most serious of which is a reaction termed anaphylactic shock. This allergic reaction occurs in approximately 1 percent of cases and is five to ten times more prevalent in female patients than in males. In anaphylactic shock the body experiences a severe reaction that affects practically every vital organ. The result can be death within minutes. However, since this serious reaction is known to be a potential hazard with intradiskal therapy, doctors have the medications, equipment, and life-saving devices at hand when performing chemonucleolysis. When properly treated in a timely fashion, anaphylactic shock is seldom fatal. Less severe but more frequently encountered adverse reactions include back pain and muscle spasms, rash, and generalized swelling.

Surgery has a place, but a very limited one, in treating back pain. Although there remains the common notion that if there is really to be any hope for definitive relief of the pain, surgery must be performed eventually and everything else is mere palliation, this idea is far from valid. In most patients with back pain, not only would surgery be useless in relieving the pain, but it could do further damage and cause increased pain. In those few cases where a back operation is indicated, surgery is an effective and useful treatment technique. But let the buyer beware—surgery is not a cure-all.

THE TOLLISON PROGRAM

We have now looked at the history of back pain, studied why backs ache, and reviewed traditional medical treatments for the painful back. If you are a victim of chronic back pain, perhaps you have tried many of the treatments described but with little relief.

If your back has continued to hurt despite the best efforts of modern medical care, do not despair. At our PAIN THERAPY CENTERS programs, the Tollison Program for back pain relief has been used with thousands of back pain victims, and with impressive results.

The remainder of this book will outline components of the Tollison Program for pain relief. Many of the treatments are part of the clinical regimen offered at our centers. Read this section carefully and discuss the treatment program with your doctor. You may find that the Tollison Program can make a significant difference in reducing your pain and helping you live a more enjoyable and productive life.

9

PHYSICAL EXERCISE: WHAT YOU DON'T USE, YOU LOSE

The first component of the Tollison Program for relieving chronic back pain is a sound, regular, and specialized program of physical exercise. And before you protest that there is no way you can exercise when the mere act of walking and bending causes increased pain, give me an opportunity to explain.

Physical exercise occupies a special and important place in the program because chronic back pain is a *psychobiological* problem. In fact, the entire program is based on the evidence that chronic back pain has both physical and emotional components. Your back begins to ache and common sense, as well as many physicians, tell you to go home, be less active, take it easy, and perhaps go to bed and take muscle relaxant medications. This advice is fine for a day or two, but a week later your back continues to hurt so you remain less physically active. A month or so later, you feel a bit better, as long as you do little more than eat, sleep, and swallow medication. But take a walk around the block, cut the grass, or clean the house, and here comes the pain again.

So what do you do? There are several alternatives, but most back victims again curtail their physical activities, take more pain pills, and become increasingly irritated and frustrated over the fact that the back is taking so long to heal.

Give physical inactivity and mounting emotional distress a few more weeks to develop, and you are on your way to becoming another statistic in the escalating number of chronic back pain victims.

Furthermore, you have also joined the casualty ranks of *hypokinesis*.

Hypokinesis, derived from the Greek *hypo* (under) and *kinesis* (motion), describes the state of decreased physical activity. Hypokinesis can affect anyone, but particularly chronic back victims whose movement often causes pain. When we are less physically active, our muscles lose strength and endurance and will eventually shrink, contract, and tighten. Furthermore, muscles that are underused do not make proper use of oxygen and soon lose their tone. Fatty deposits can accumulate under the skin and the skin will stretch and dimple. Muscles fatigue easily and you soon feel drained, tired, and depressed. Future attempts to become more physically active are discouraged because movement forces deconditioned and tightened muscles to exceed their weakened capacity, which further increases pain and misery.

And if that is not enough, hypokinesis can cause even greater physical problems. Each year millions of individuals suffer the added consequences of chronic hypokinesis. One out of three men has a heart attack by the age of 60. Obesity, stroke, lack of productivity, shortness of breath, circulatory problems, chronic fatigue, depression, and even advanced aging are also thought to be associated with hypokinesis.

SOME BENEFITS OF EXERCISE

But it is never too late to take the first step toward physical fitness, improved general health, and back pain relief. All it involves is: (1) a commitment on your part to invest the time and effort required to benefit from a program of physical reconditioning, (2) medical clearance and agreement from your physician, and (3) knowledge gained from this chapter on effective stretching, strengthening, and conditioning exercises. Consider the payoff from your investment.

The Muscles

With proper physical exercise, weak, tired, and tight muscles gradually stretch and become stronger. Since weak and contracted back and abdominal muscles frequently play a major role in chronic back pain, this is good news for the person who is tired of suffering.

With regular exercise changes occur within the cells of our muscles. And as cells change, so do muscle fibers. Muscle contraction is both fast and stronger, which requires less exertion on your part and builds stamina. Because the muscle fibers don't fatigue as easily, endurance is increased, and you experience less fatigue and have more energy. In addition, tight and painful back muscles that, like a rope, refuse to stretch will gradually become more like a rubber band and your flexibility and range of motion will increase. Furthermore, muscles that respond to stress, irritation, and anxiety by tensing, tightening, and causing increased pain are prone to remain limber and loose and you are likely to enjoy improved sleep and a comforting sense of well-being.

The Mind

Exercise, it seems, is often an effective and healthy nonchemical tranquilizer. In a study conducted at Purdue University in Lafayette, Ind., 60 middle-aged faculty and staff members, all of them employed in sedentary jobs, participated in a four-month exercise program. Their personalities were evaluated both before and after the program, using a variety of psychological tests. As they became better conditioned physically, the subjects were found to become more emotionally stable, more self-sufficient, more imaginative, and more confident.

Dr. Richard Driscoll of Eastern State Psychiatric Hospital in Knoxville, Tenn., also found that regular exercise makes people less anxious, particularly if they think pleasant thoughts during the workout. Dr. Michael B. Mock of the National Heart, Lung and Blood Institute reports that exercise has been found to counteract depressed feelings by increasing one's feeling of self-esteem and independence.

Dr. John Griest of the University of Wisconsin recently reported some rather startling investigative results. Dr. Griest assigned patients suffering from depression to either a ten-week exercise program or ten weeks of psychotherapy. The results of his study suggest that the exercise program was more effective in alleviating depression. While there are methodological flaws in some of the research cited, the general suggestion is clear: A regular program of exercise has a positive effect on our personalities.

Dr. Hans Selye of the University of Montreal has been studying stress for four decades. He believes that each of us possesses at birth a given amount of what he calls adaptation energy. When that energy is depleted, we experience a mental or physical breakdown. One way to avoid such a breakdown is by deliberately directing stress at varying body systems. Dr. Selye believes that a voluntary change of activity is as good as, or even better than, rest. For example, when fatigued at the end of a long, tough day at the office, it is better to exercise rigorously for 30 minutes than to take a short nap. Substituting demands on our musculature for those previously made on the intellect not only gives our brain a rest, but it helps to relax the body as well. Dr. Selye believes that stress on one body system helps to relax another and this is good news for back pain victims!

The Nerves

Nerves benefit from physical conditioning by becoming better at transmitting electrochemical impulses and activating more muscle fibers, thereby increasing strength. Furthermore, as reflexes replace voluntary actions, movement becomes more efficient. Wasteful muscular contractions become fewer, unneeded muscles relax more fully, and movement is simplified. In short, the body becomes a more finely tuned and productive machine.

The Blood

Embraced by hemoglobin, blood travels throughout our bodies delivering oxygen to the muscles. To increase the blood's efficiency as exercise begins, fluid leaves the bloodstream and fills small cavities between muscle cells. This serves two important purposes. First, the muscles work more smoothly and easily when bathed in fluid; second, the blood's hemoglobin concentration rises, allowing a given volume of blood to transport more oxygen than usual.

With a regular program of physical conditioning and exercise, an important change takes place in the blood. The body, in effect learning to expect its blood volume to be periodically lowered, increases its supply; consequently, when fluid leaves the bloodstream at the onset of exercise, a larger quantity remains to carry out essential tasks.

With a consistent program of exercise, the composition of the blood is changed in still other ways. For example, its clotting ability is enhanced. Since clots, once formed, must be dissolved, the enzyme called fibrinolysin appears in greater quantities. At the same time, certain lipids, such as the types of cholesterol and triglycerides associated with heart disease, become less concentrated in the blood.

The Heart

Few effects of physical conditioning have been more thoroughly documented than those that occur within the heart. Research has demonstrated that with proper conditioning the heart becomes a distinctly more efficient instrument, capable of doing more while working less. One of the most fundamental changes that takes place is the lengthening of the heart muscle fibers; a similar process occurs in the lengthening of leg muscles when we do stretching exercises. Longer fibers allow the heart's chambers to pump more blood with each contraction. As a result the heart rate slows as the heart becomes more efficient. In addition, blood pressure during rest is usually reduced. Since high blood pressure is known to contribute to heart attacks, a lowering of the pressure is a welcome benefit of exercise.

We have briefly reviewed just a few of the many advantages of a proper program of physical conditioning. While no unequivocal scientific data exist to date, most scientists believe that proper physical conditioning prolongs life. Even if the lifespan is not expanded, there is little argument that the quality of life is enhanced by exercise. Physical conditioning relieves pain and stress, relaxes tense muscles, and improves endurance and vascular blood flow—all of which are usually associated in some way with chronic back pain.

A GUIDE FOR RECONDITIONING THE BACK AND BODY

At our Pain Therapy Centers,™ we firmly believe that a specialized, daily program of physical exercise can make a significant difference in the intensity of pain that most back victims suffer. Although you may notice increased discomfort during the first two exercise program due to muscle soreness and fatigue, in most cases this slight increase in discomfort is no cause for alarm. Keep in mind that there is a major difference between hurt and damage. The exercise component at our centers may cause some initial increased hurt, but is designed to avoid damage. It is always a good idea to consult a physician prior to beginning an exercise program, and it is *particularly significant for chronic back pain victims!* Take this book to your doctor to review the outlined exercises before you begin your program.

With your physician's approval, it's time to take charge of your back pain by beginning a regular exercise program. The exercises illustrated and discussed throughout the remainder of this chapter are specifically designed for back pain victims and are divided into three major sections: stretching, strengthening, and conditioning. Familiarize yourself with the entire program before beginning.

It is important to be realistic in your anticipation of progress. Do not set goals for distance, time, and endurance, but rather exercise at a leisurely pace and let progress occur naturally. Expectations are not conducive to relaxation and can make your reconditioning program stressful and laborious. Your aim is not to enter the Olympics, but to ease your back discomfort and improve your general health. Design your exercise program to be relaxing and enjoyable. Your back and your body will thank you!

STRETCHING EXERCISES

The object of stretching exercises is *gradually* to stretch muscles and body parts that have tightened and shortened due to hypokinesis or physical inactivity. You will likely feel the muscles pulling and stretching as you perform these exercises. With repeated and con-sistent exercise, your muscles, which may initially feel like ropes, will gradually stretch and your back misery should begin to decrease. Always start your daily exercise program with the stretching exercises before proceeding to strengthening and conditioning exercises.

Lateral Arm Swing

The lateral arm swing is performed by standing with your feet slightly apart and your arms straight out by your sides as shown. Now swing your arms out in front of you and let them cross. Return your arms to the original position and then continue swinging them

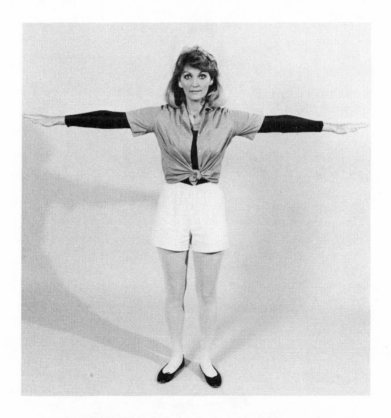

Photographs 9-1 and 9-2—The Lateral Arm Swing will stretch the muscles in your upper arms, upper back, and shoulders.

back and forth. This exercise will stretch the muscles in your upper arms, upper back, and shoulders. Begin with leisurely swings and gradually increase the intensity of your efforts. Let your endurance build naturally.

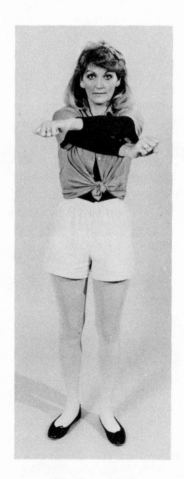

Photograph 9-2

Vertical Arm Swing

Begin this exercise by letting your arms hang by your sides. Now swing one arm over your head. Next switch the position of your arms and keep swinging in a constant rhythmic motion. The vertical arm swing stretches the muscles in the upper back, shoulders, and neck that frequently tighten when we are tense, stressed, or in pain.

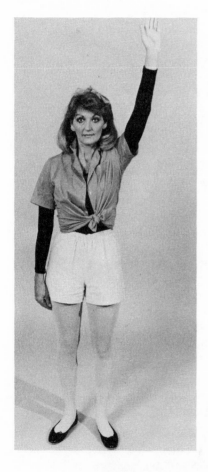 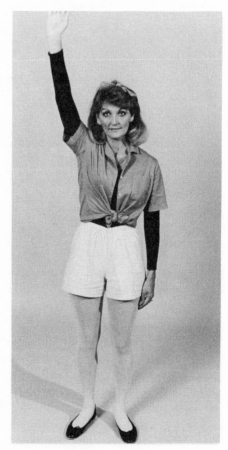

Photographs 9-3 and 9-4—The Vertical Arm Swing can help stretch and relax painfully tight muscles in the upper back, neck, and shoulders.

Back Arches

Begin this exercise by leaning against a wall with your feet approximately six inches from the wall. Push your arms and shoulders back against the wall, stretching the muscles in the upper back, shoulders, and neck, similar to the military "attention!" posture. As you do this, *slightly* arch your back and hold this position for about ten seconds before relaxing. Now relax for ten seconds, and repeat. Repetitions of this exercise should gradually increase at a natural pace.

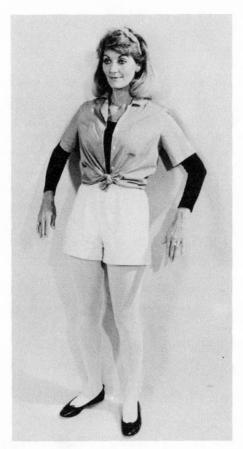

Photograph 9-5—Hold the military "Attention!" posture for about 10 seconds before relaxing and work toward increasing your repetitions of this important exercise.

Calf and Heel Cord Stretch

Stand with your feet between one and two feet from the wall and your arms in front with your hands on the wall about the height of your shoulders. Now hold your stomach in as you lean into the wall. Do not arch your back. Make sure that your feet stay flat on the floor and your knees are straight. Hold the stretch for ten seconds, then return to the original position. Repeat the exercise and let your repetitions gradually increase. This exercise will stretch the muscles in the calves as well as the heel cord (Achilles tendon) that runs up the back of the heel.

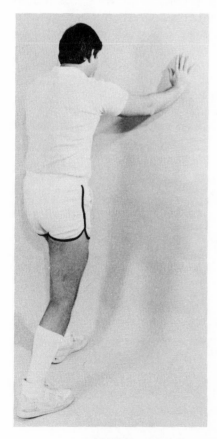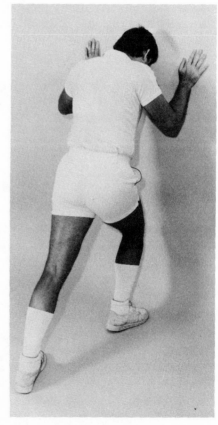

Photographs 9-6 and 9-7—The Calf and Heel Cord Stretch will assist in reconditioning muscles in the calves as well as the heel cord that usually tighten in response to prolonged disease.

Hamstring Stretch

Perform the hamstring stretch by resting your weight on one arm on the armrest of a chair while standing at the side of the chair. Then walk slowly toward the chair. Move your feet forward until your toes are close to the leg of the chair. Be sure that you bend your body at the hips and keep your back straight, and also that you continue resting your upper body weight on your arm. You should feel the stretch of your hamstring muscles. These are the muscles that go up the back of each leg. You can further stretch these muscles by pulling your toes up toward the head, and even more by also raising your leg out to the side of the chair with your toes pulled up. Work your way up by gradually bending over and getting your head closer to the seat of the chair. Be sure to work gradually!

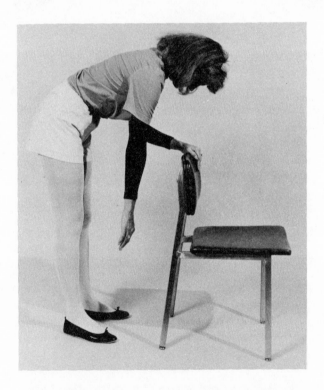

Photograph 9-8—Hamstring tightness is commonly associated with chronic back pain. The Hamstring Stretch can help loosen tight muscles.

Bend Sitting

This exercise should be performed while sitting in a straight chair with your feet apart. Rest most of your upper body weight on one knee by propping an elbow on your knee. Then gradually try to touch the floor with your other hand. Don't force yourself, but swing your arm from front to back between your legs. Before long you'll be able to put your hands flat on the floor. Use the opposite arm each time you do the exercise. Bend sitting will help stretch the muscles in the shoulders, or back, and in the back of your legs.

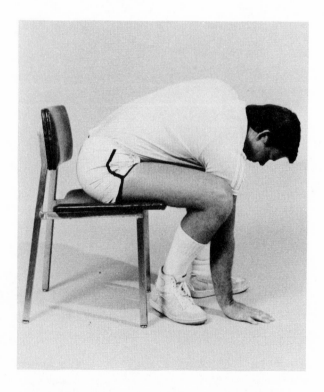

Photograph 9-9—Always rest your upper body weight on one knee to avoid straining the muscles in the lower back.

Knee–Chest Stretch

For the knee-chest exercise, lie on your back and raise your knees until you can grasp your right knee with your right hand and your left knee with your left hand. Keep your knees apart and gradually pull both of them toward your chest. Hold this position for ten seconds. Now slowly go back to your original position, relax, and repeat. This exercise will stretch the muscles in your lower back and buttocks.

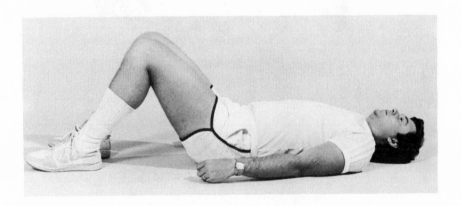

Photographs 9-10, 9-11 and 9-12—The Knee-Chest Stretch will gradually stretch tight and painful muscles in the lower back.

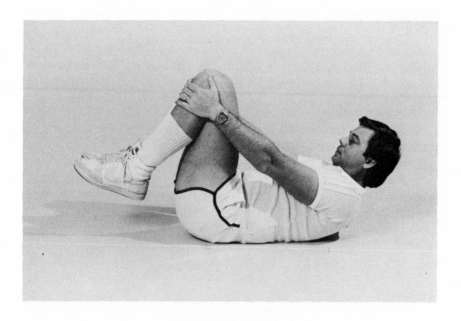

Photograph 9-11

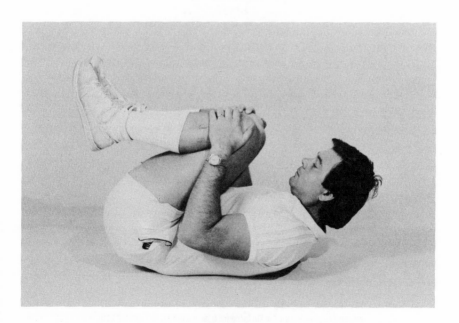

Photograph 9-12

Pectoral Stretch

Sit in a straight chair and place your hands behind your neck, interlacing the fingers. Now bring your elbows as far back as you can and hold for a count of five. Return to your starting position, relax, and repeat. Let the repetitions build gradually and naturally.

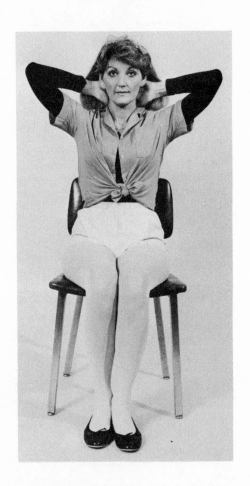

Photograph 9-13—Repetitions of all exercises, including the Pectoral Stretch, should build gradually and naturally.

STRENGTHENING EXERCISES

The object of strengthening exercises is *gradually* to strengthen muscles that have weakened due to chronic pain and hypokinesis. It is important that once you start an exercise program, you continue it every day. Keep in mind that the exercises outlined may cause initial muscle stiffness and soreness, but there is a major difference between hurt and damage. If you begin your exercise program in a wise and gradual fashion but find that the exercises create severe pain, consult your physician. You can generally minimize initial discomfort by beginning your program with slow, gentle exercises and gradually easing into a more strenuous program.

Curl-Ups

Curl-ups are a substitution for sit-ups. Unlike sit-ups, they can strengthen your stomach muscles without your running the risk of pulling or injuring your back. Curl-ups are done by lying on your back with your lower legs and feet resting on a small stool. Reach toward your knees with your hands, then raise your head and then your shoulders while curling your upper body forward. Now slowly return to your original position, rest, and repeat. There is no need to sit up any further than is necessary to touch your knees. Sitting up further than this increases the amount of stress and strain placed on your lower back and causes unnecessary risk.

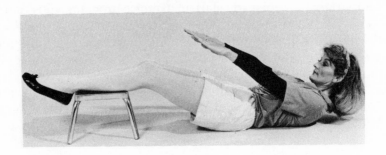

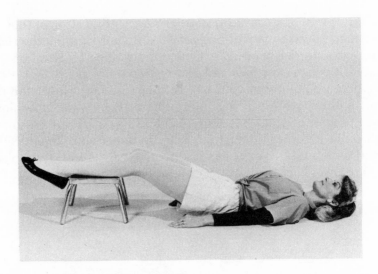

Photographs 9-14 and 9-15—Curl-ups are a safe and effective substitute for sit-ups.

Wall Slide Hold

Begin this exercise by standing with your back and shoulders against a wall and your feet 18 to 24 inches from the wall. Slowly slide your back and hips down the wall until you are sitting in an imaginary chair. Hold this position for several minutes, or until you are fatigued. If needed, stand up and rest a moment before returning to the sitting position. Using the exercise quota system explained in Chapter 15, add five or ten seconds every other day until you can hold the wall-slide for four to five minutes. This exercise is excellent for strengthening the leg muscles, which are very important in lifting, proper body mechanics, and proper back care.

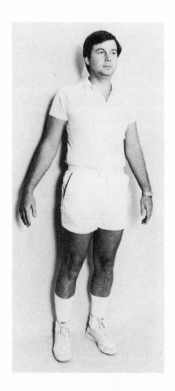 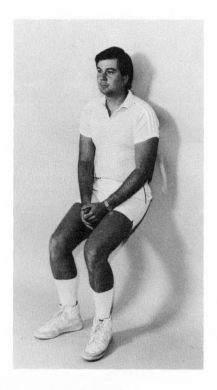

Photographs 9-16 and 9-17—The Wall Slide Hold can be practiced almost anywhere. Remember that strong legs are important in proper spinal care.

Pelvic Tilt

To perform the pelvic tilt, lie on your back with your knees bent and your feet flat on the floor. With your arms lying by your side, push the small of your back down into the floor. At the same time, pinch your buttocks together and pull your stomach in. Make sure your back is flat against the floor and do *not* lift your buttocks from the floor. The pelvic tilt exercise will decrease the amount of stress on your back, and at the same time strengthen the muscles in your stomach and buttocks.

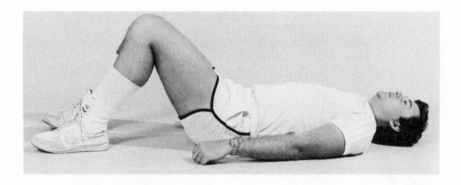

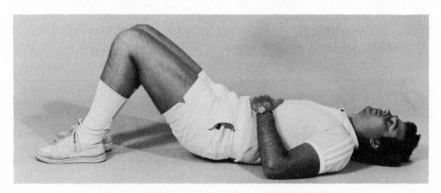

Photographs 9-18 and 9-19—Try to get into a Pelvic Tilt habit. After sufficient practice, the Pelvic Tilt can be used when standing and walking to stabilize the spine and decrease spinal stress.

Upper Back

For this exercise lie on your stomach with your arms at your sides. While you exhale raise your shoulders and chest off the floor. Hold this position for a count of six and then return to the starting position, relax, and repeat. This exercise will strengthen the muscles in your upper back and across your shoulders. Add to your repetitions gradually.

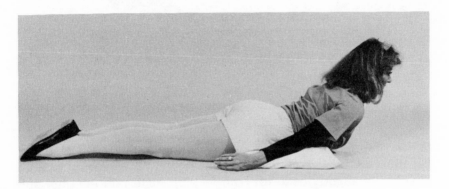

Photograph 9-20—Muscular strength and flexibility are both important in the care of a painful back.

Single Leg Raise

This exercise is designed to strengthen the muscles in your lower back and abdomen, both of which are important in proper back care. Lie on your back with a pillow under your hips and your arms under your head. Raise one leg and hold for a count of five, then lower the leg and relax. Repeat with the other leg. Repetitions should increase as your physical conditioning improves. After prolonged physical inactivity, this exercise may at first seem difficult. Start slow and easy, and build your strength and stamina.

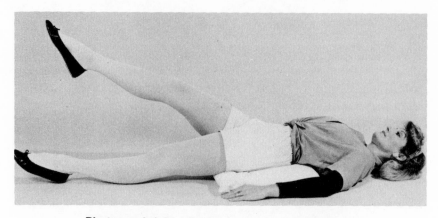

Photograph 9-21—Remember to start your exercise program slow and easy and build your muscular strength in the stomach and back with the Single Leg Raise.

Hip Flexor

The hip flexor is designed to strengthen both the stomach and hip muscles. Lie flat on the floor with your arms to your sides. With knees only slightly bent, lift both feet ten inches off the floor and hold for ten seconds. Then return, relax, and repeat. If raising both legs creates too great a strain, start by alternating one leg at a time until your strength increases.

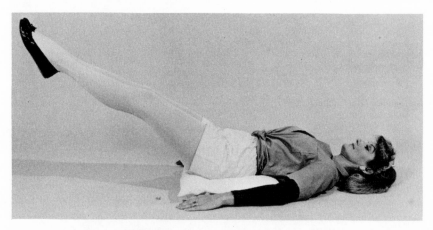

Photograph 9-22—If raising both legs is too difficult, start out by alternating one leg at a time.

CONDITIONING EXERCISES

After stretching and strengthening, reconditioning your back and body to combat the effects of hypokinesis is critical. A limber, strong, and conditioned back is almost guaranteed to hurt less, and a properly conditioned body will have more energy, vitality, and stamina. Conditioning exercises can have a positive effect on your entire body and mind and the "winners" in the battle against chronic back pain will use this knowledge to their advantage.

There are numerous appropriate and effective conditioning exercises. But few of them can match the overall benefit of a program of regular walking.

Walking

Walking is considered by many experts to be the most efficient exercise for improving overall fitness and physical conditioning. It uses more muscles than other forms of exercise in a continuous, uniform action, and it remains accessible to us throughout life. Walking is often an integral part of medical programs designed to prevent heart-related diseases and to rehabilitate those already suffering heart trouble. Furthermore, a regular program of walking is known to partially combat the effects of hypokinesis. Walking is a major part of the Tollison program for back pain relief.

The first step in a successful conditioning program is to find the walking routine that is best suited to your current physical condition. If back pain has limited your tolerance for prolonged walking, it is wise to start slowly and gradually build as your stamina and strength increase.

Strolling about one mile per hour is perhaps the slowest form of walking, but do not underestimate its value. Even prolonged strolling for several hours can add extra miles of needed physical exercise. However, strolling will benefit you more in terms of limbering tight muscles than actual body conditioning. To receive the value of physical conditioning, it is necessary gradually to work your way through strolling to normal or aerobic walking.

Normal walking usually averages about three miles per hour and, depending on the distance walked, can be of conditioning benefit. Take every opportunity to walk, whether down the street to the post office or around the block for exercise. As you steadily increase your time and distance, calories will burn, muscles will strengthen and limber, and needed oxygen will flow freely to your muscles and brain.

Aerobic walking is the most advanced form of walking performed with speed, duration, and effort to exercise the heart, lungs, back, and entire body. Most forms of walking can be converted to aerobic exercise simply by maintaining a rapid pace, increasing the movement of your arms, or climbing an incline. Few chronic back pain victims can or should begin their reconditioning exercise program with aerobic walking and some may never be able to build to this advanced form. While aerobic walking is excellent full-body exercise, our primary goal is to minimize your back discomfort. The most important parts of reconditioning walking are the regularity of exercise and a slow and gradual increase in speed and duration. Back pain "winners" neither underdo nor overdo, but give thought to their exercise program and maintain a gradually increasing effort.

Be wise—exercise!

In summary, physical exercise is the first part of the Tollison Program for back pain relief. But exercise is certainly not the only part of our program, nor is it necessarily the most significant part. The program is a psychobiological, multifaceted program of back care of which physical exercise is but one, albeit important, part. Relaxation training is explained in the next chapter, and the remainder of this book is devoted to the explanation and illustration of other vital components. Remember that the Tollison Program is not "bandaid therapy" or a "quick fix," but a lifetime recipe for back pain relief composed of many ingredients.

Continue reading, studying, and practicing!

10

RELAXATION TRAINING

Most of us live a pressure cooker existence. There are bills to be paid, children to be cared for, marital and spousal demands, less-than-satisfying jobs, checkbooks to be balanced, taxes to be paid, traffic to be fought, and so on. Little wonder that we long for a simpler life; to transform ourselves somehow to a less stressful place in time or to live, say, like a cat.

When a cat is not disturbed, it is perfectly at ease. Every muscle is supple and relaxed. Yet when the cat becomes irritated or angered, you can watch it become tense before your eyes. It spits and hisses; it arches its back and prepares to fight or to flee. When the irritability reaches a certain point, the cat either attacks or runs away. In either case it carries out a physical response. The cat does not sit and stew as we do. It responds physically, and afterward returns to a state of ease and relaxation.

Unfortunately contemporary man and woman have a similar physiological structure. When we are faced with a stressful situation, our bodies involuntarily prepare to take action. But unlike a cat, we seldom fight or flee. The rules of civilized society discourage these options, and usually we do nothing but sit and seethe. This constant suppression of a natural physical response puts an unnatural strain on our system. And like any system strained beyond its capabilities, something is going to give. In the case of modern man and woman, we pay the price with our health.

Stress is increasingly recognized by health care professionals as an "epidemic" and a major contributing factor in a variety of physical and psychological disorders. A partial listing of recognized stress-related disorders includes chronic pain, headaches, back pain, stomach distress, high blood pressure, heart problems, irritability, asthma, anxiety, temper outbursts, employee absenteeism, lost productivity, marital discord, chronic fatigue, and sexual dysfunction. In fact, the American Academy of Family Physicians states that two-thirds of office visits to family doctors are prompted by stress-related symptoms. At the same time, leaders of industry have become alarmed by the enormous cost of stress symptoms, which is estimated at between $50 and $75 billion annually, or more than $750 for every U.S. worker. The national stress epidemic is further evidenced by the fact that the three best-selling prescription drugs in this country are an ulcer medication (Tagamet), a drug to control high blood pressure (Inderal), and a tranquilizer (Valium).

What have the damaging effects of stress to do with your aching back? The answer: a great deal more than perhaps you ever realized. We discussed in earlier chapters the fact that stress, tension, and anxiety cause generalized muscle tension throughout the body. We also know that prolonged muscle tension depletes the muscles of oxygen and blood, thereby allowing a build-up of toxins that may result in the sensation we know as pain (see Chapter 3, Figure 3-1). The build-up of stress and muscle tension with resultant back pain is best exemplified by two individuals whom we will call Scott and Judy.

Scott is a bigamist, but not the kind anyone, especially his legal wife, can do anything about. Why? Because Scott is a corporate bigamist—someone married to his job as well as to his wife. And, if you ask his wife, Scott takes the contract he signed with his employer much more seriously than the vows he made to her on their wedding day.

If you don't want to use fancy names, you can call Scott a workaholic. He's at the office each day at 7 a.m. to start his day of meetings, conferences, problem solving, budget reports, and stacks of paper work. The telephone rings constantly and he gulps down cups of coffee between outbursts of irritation over the calls. Fourteen hours later Scott packs his briefcase with paper work to take home and heads for the door. His back aches and he stops at the water fountain to swallow a few more pain pills to get him through the night. Two hours later Scott takes a tranquilizer to help him unwind from the hectic day and help him sleep.

Scott is an emotional wreck—an obsessed, anxious, driven soul who lives each day as if there were no tomorrow. His heart races and his blood pressure soars, his stomach pours out ulcer-causing acid and his heart works overtime to pump blood through vessels constricted by stress and anxiety. His back aches from generalized muscular tension and he is miserable. Scott finally takes the time to visit his doctor, but only because he wants pain pills to ease his back misery so that he can keep going. His doctor talks to him about stress, tension, and pain, but Scott doesn't listen. He fails to see the connection between his life-style and back pain because he doesn't listen to the doctor. Scott is too busy creating his own back pain through uncontrolled tension, stress, and anxiety to realize what he is doing.

Judy is a good wife, a loving mother to two young children, and a valued employee at a local factory. She and her husband have worked hard to provide for themselves and are proud of their new home, car, and boat. To her friends Judy is a model of success—good job, loving family, new home, and active in the church and her son's peewee baseball league.

But one day everything changes. While bending to lift a box from the floor, Judy feels a sudden snap in her back and pain suddenly engulfs her body. Unable to straighten up, she falls to the floor in excrutiating pain.

Judy's doctor diagnoses a severe muscular and ligament strain of the lower back and sends her home to stay in bed for three weeks. Judy panics. Who will care for her husband and children? What about her job? Isn't there some pill that the doctor can give her that will allow her to continue her routine?

Because the severity of pain leaves her no choice, Judy follows her doctor's advice. But rather than relaxing and resting in bed, Judy worries. What if she doesn't get better? Are the children eating properly without her preparing the meals? How will her husband react to the forced cancellation of their planned weekend boating trips? And the more Judy worries, the more her back aches.

Three weeks later Judy returns to her doctor unimproved. Not only does she continue suffering severe back pain, but now feels stiff and sore all over and also complains of daily headaches. The doctor hospitalizes Judy for a myelogram and CT scan (Chapter 5) but the diagnosis is unchanged. According to the objective medical evidence, Judy should be improving rather than deteriorating into a web of pain and worry.

One month later, Judy is worse than ever. She can hardly move because of her severe pain and spends most of her time in bed. She obsesses over mounting bills and fears losing their new home. Her young children miss their mother and Judy feels increasingly guilty over missed meals and baseball games. She is upset, worried, tense, and nervous, and her back hurts all the more.

Six months later, Judy is a victim of the "pain–tension cycle" and is firmly trapped in the clutches of chronic back pain. The more she can't do, the more tense and worried she becomes. And the more tense and worried she becomes, the more she can't do. Judy is trapped in a vicious cycle of pain, suffering, and disability caused, in large part, by her inability to relax.

Chronic anxiety and stress are most commonly, as illustrated by our story of Scott, a subtle and insidious parasite with no identifiable onset. It slowly drains us of our natural physiological and psychological resiliency. It can also lower our resistence and set the stage for the development of numerous physical disorders, including chronic back pain. Yet the people most controlled by chronic stress and tension are usually the last to recognize their affliction. In treating thousands of patients at our centers, it has been my experience that suggesting to individuals such as Scott that chronic stress and muscular tension are a major cause of back pain is almost guaranteed to elicit a response of total surprise and disbelief. When I follow with an explanation of the importance of relaxation skills to control their pain, some pain victims shake their heads in disbelief and go off to find another doctor. A few of these sufferers will pause at the door and leave me with their opinion that "nothing could be that easy" before exiting. Those individuals who suffer chronic stress, tension, and back pain and who accept my explanation of the pain–tension cycle as the cause of their pain are generally well pleased with the pain relief that results from daily practice of relaxation training.

Do you suffer chronic or excessive stress and anxiety? Do you feel that there is a chance your back pain could be the result of stress and tension? Before you answer remember that chronic stress and tension may be very much a part of your life although you don't feel particularly tense or nervous. Take five minutes to complete the screening inventory in Table 10-1. This inventory has *not* been subjected to statistical reliability and validity studies and is intended only to offer a small sampling of traits and symptoms generally believed to be associated with chronic stress and tension.

Back pain victims such as Judy represent another important way in which tension and anxiety play a significant role in chronic back pain. Unlike Scott, Judy did not suffer chronic stress and tension before her back injury. But her back injury altered her life both physiologically and psychologically. Physiologically Judy suffered intense pain, which, according to our pain–tension cycle, creates

TABLE 10-1
STRESS AND TENSION SCREENING INVENTORY

This inventory is intended only to offer a sampling of traits and symptoms often associated with chronic stress and tension.

DIRECTIONS: Read each statement carefully and answer TRUE or FALSE as the statement applies to your life.

1. I spend less than five hours each week participating in hobbies that are totally unrelated to my work.
2. I worry too much.
3. Often I feel a tightness in my neck and shoulders.
4. I tend to eat when I'm uptight or worried.
5. My back feels tight and sore at the end of the day.
6. I frequently have difficulty falling asleep.
7. I sometimes drink alcohol to unwind.
8. There is at least one person in my family whom I consider overly nervous.
9. I feel tense much of the time.
10. I often have sweaty palms or perspire excessively.
11. I have more than one headache per month.
12. I feel weak and tired much of the time.
13. I consider myself a nervous person.
14. I am somewhat superstitious.
15. I am easily awakened by noise.
16. My neck and shoulder muscles are sometimes sore and tender.
17. I often find it difficult to unwind and feel totally relaxed and peaceful.
18. I have diarrhea or indigestion more than twice a month.
19. I am sometimes afraid of losing control of myself.
20. I need to lose weight.
21. Others probably consider me a nervous person.
22. I smoke cigarettes (cigar, pipe).
23. I often seem weak and seem to tire more easily than others.
24. I am easily startled by loud noises.
25. Often I feel as if there were a tight band around my head.
26. I eat faster than most people.
27. I take medication for my nerves (even occasionally).

Males
1. I often ejaculate too quickly during sexual intercourse.
2. I have difficulty achieving an erection sufficient for intercourse more than once per month.
3. I often have difficulty ejaculating during intercourse.

Females
1. I frequently have difficulty achieving orgasm during intercourse.
2. Often I am so tense that intercourse is painful or unpleasant.
3. The thought of sexual intercourse is frequently an unpleasant thought that I try to push from my mind.

Scoring: Positive responses (TRUE) to five or more of the above statements may indicate that you are more anxious than need be.

prolonged muscular tension, which creates more pain, which creates more muscular tension, which creates even more pain, and so on. If that were not enough, Judy also suffered a number of marked changes in life-style. In recent years some very important research has been conducted on identifying certain events commonly encountered in our lives and the impact of these events in creating tension and anxiety. One such research effort was conducted by T. H. Holmes and R. H. Rahe, who first published their work for the scientific community and later for the general public in a 1973 *New York Times* article. According to these investigators, changes in our lives cause tension and anxiety, which can be measured in what they term "life-change units." Their research suggests that the accumulation of over 200 life-change units in a year is associated with problem tension, nervousness, anxiety, and most important, a high incidence of physical illness.

According to the authors, the tension and anxiety resulting from a traumatic life change frequently sets the stage for the onset of disease involving any organ system in the body and with any degree of severity. This tension-, anxiety-, or stress-related illness may be emotional turmoil with no organic disease, exacerbation of an existing but previously tolerated physical illness, new organic disease, or a combination of any of the foregoing. In Judy's case the combination of back pain and resulting muscular tension, together with the life changes, stress, and further muscular tension and pain, was simply more than she could handle. She had a physical injury that was compounded and complicated by physiological and psychological reactions that combined to result in suffering and disability. After her injury Judy fell victim to the pain–tension cycle.

LEARNING TO "REALLY" RELAX

Whether our pain is similar to Scott's or to Judy's, to break the powerful influence that stress and muscle tension have on back pain requires that we learn to relax. By relaxing I don't mean kicking off your shoes and falling asleep during a favorite television show or lazily lounging around in the back yard. To neutralize the powerful influence of chronic muscular tension in back pain requires an antidote equally as powerful. It requires (1) a system of total body relaxation, (2) an organized means of implementation, (3) a research-

TABLE 10-2
THE STRESS OF ADJUSTING TO CHANGE—"LIFE-CHANGE UNITS"

Accumulation of over 200 "life change units" in a
year is believed to be associated with problem
tension, nervousness, and a high incidence of
physical illness.

1.	Death of spouse	100
2.	Divorce	73
3.	Marital separation	63
4.	Jail term	63
5.	Death of close family member	63
6.	Personal injury or illness	53
7.	Marriage	50
8.	Fired from job	47
9.	Marital reconciliation	45
10.	Retirement	45
11.	Change in health of family member	44
12.	Pregnancy	40
13.	Sex difficulties	39
14.	Gain of new family member	39
15.	Business readjustment	39
16.	Change in financial state	38
17.	Death of close friend	37
18.	Change to different line of work	36
19.	Change in number of arguments with spouse	35
20.	Mortgage over $10,000	31
21.	Foreclosure of mortgage or loan	30
22.	Change in responsibilities at work	29
23.	Son or daughter leaving home	29
24.	Trouble with inlaws	29
25.	Outstanding personal achievement	28
26.	Spouse begins or stops work	26
27.	Begin or end school	26
28.	Change in living conditions	25
29.	Revision of personal habits	24
30.	Trouble with boss	23
31.	Change in work hours or conditions	20
32.	Change in residence	20
33.	Change in schools	20
34.	Change in recreation	19
35.	Change in church activities	19
36.	Change in social activities	18
37.	Mortgage or loan less than $10,000	17
38.	Change in sleeping habits	16
39.	Change in number of family get-togethers	15
40.	Change in eating habits	15
41.	Vacation	13
42.	Christmas	12
43.	Minor violation of the law	11

Holmes, T. H., and Rahe, R. H., *The New York Times*, June 10, 1973, Reprinted with
permission.

based effective technique, and (4) a structured schedule of practice.

For our purposes we can consider relaxation as the opposite of tension. Most people readily assume that one flourishes in the absence of the other; that is, if you are not tense, you must be relaxed. Unfortunately the human body doesn't function that simply. If you consider relaxation positioned on one end of a continuum and tension on the other, there is a huge gray area in between where we all exist most of the time. A typical day may have some moments of tension and some of relaxation but we usually exist in a kind of psychic limbo. Yet often tension is building within us. Stimuli too small to be consciously registered are tightening our muscles, aggravating our nerves, and constricting our blood vessels. Back pain is causing our muscles to tighten, which increases our pain and further muscle contraction in spasm. By the end of the day, we are incapacitated by back discomfort and hurting too badly to sleep.

Relaxation cannot build in our bodies as we go through a routine day because so much stress and tension exist in our lives. To combat the negative effects, we must learn to relax. Simply defined, relaxation is the absence of mental and physical stress, which is achieved when the body is in equilibrium and the mind is unhampered by anxiety. It is physiologically impossible and psychologically impractical for an individual always to be relaxed, since the mind thrives on a certain amount of controlled, creative turbulence. It is, however, feasible for each of us to be able to control bodily processes enough to regulate the energy and excitation flow of the system.

The ability to relax can have a dramatic effect on the body. Amazing physiological changes occur in the relaxed body; heartbeat and respiration slow, and the quality of electrical waves in the brain changes. Alpha waves, which can be recorded from the brain during peaceful, tranquil moments when the eyes are closed, become more numerous. Research conducted at the Johns Hopkins Clinic in Baltimore suggests that using biofeedback to teach subjects to increase the percentage of alpha waves from the brain may reduce headache frequency. Muscles also loosen and lengthen during relaxation, which reduces back pain.

Physiological relaxation most often leads to cognitive or psychological relaxation. The emotions are tranquil, and a feeling of peace prevails. Western scientists have found that the simple process of meditation, thought by many to be a form of relaxation, can have wide-reaching physiological effects. Studies conducted on Zen monks in Japan showed that during meditation, the monks were able to decrease their consumption of oxygen and output of carbon dioxide by approximately 20 percent. Decreases in heartbeat and respiration have also been observed in yoga practitioners. All of this leads to a deceleration in metabolism, a tranquilizing of the emotional state, a reduction in tension, and a decrease in the intensity of back pain.

Deep body relaxation and control of back pain are *skills* in the same way that driving a car, playing tennis, riding a bicycle, or sewing is a learned skill. And like any skill, relaxation must be perfected through practice. Take learning to ride a bicycle. To do so requires that you first learn the parts of the vehicle—wheels, seat, handlebars, pedals, and so forth. The next step is to learn the procedure—sitting on the seat and pedaling while holding on and guiding the bicycle with the handlebars. But with this knowledge alone could someone who had never maneuvered a bicycle successfully ride? Probably not, and the reason is probably balance. To ride a bicycle necessitates a delicate job of balancing that cannot be explained, but is learned through practice.

And so it is with relaxation training. The procedure and technique will be explained in the following sections, but the real benefit must come through practice.

One particularly effective and popular relaxation technique at our centers is known as *progressive muscle relaxation*. It involves practicing exercises that mechanically manipulate the skeletal muscles of the entire body into a more deeply relaxed state. In the early 1900s, Dr. Edmond Jacobson of the Laboratory of Clinical Physiology in Chicago first outlined the principles of progressive muscle relaxation. The exercise to follow is a modification of Jacobson's technique that we have found to be effective.

As with any learned skill, practice makes perfect! With serious practice twice each day, less time is required to achieve the desired stage of deep relaxation and a decrease in back discomfort. The technique can then be used to ward off headaches, reduce stress, assist in better sleep, *and to reduce back pain!*

Procedure

1. When first learning to relax, a quiet, dimly lit place is an ideal one in which to practice.
2. Lie on your back on a carpeted floor or sit in a comfortable chair. Avoid

practicing relaxation exercises in bed since most mattresses do not provide sufficient support.

3. Try to eliminate all other competing thoughts from your mind. Relaxation exercises are intended to relax your body *and* your mind.

4. Focus all attention on the muscle group being tensed.

5. Tense muscle groups on cue. Get in the habit of following the same procedure each time you practice relaxation exercises.

6. Hold the tension and focus all attention on the build-up of tension in every muscle group for six to ten seconds.

7. Release the tension from each muscle group all at once. Do *not* gradually relax a muscle group at the end of six to ten seconds, but instead let the muscle relax suddenly, as if turning off a light switch.

8. After relaxing a muscle group, focus all of your attention on relaxation for 20 to 30 seconds. Concentrate on the different sensation between tension and relaxation.

9. Repeat for each muscle group.

10. Practice relaxation exercises at least twice daily, but the more the better!

Technique

1. Lie on your back on the floor with a pillow under your knees. Make a fist and tense the muscles of the forearm of the right hand and arm. Imagine you are holding a golf ball in the palm of the right hand and squeezing it. Relax.

2. Make a tight fist, bending the right arm at the elbow and tensing the muscles of the upper arm. Relax.

3. Make a tight fist and tense the muscles of the forearm of the left hand and arm. Imagine you are holding a golf ball in the palm of the left hand and squeezing it. Relax.

4. Make a tight fist, bending the left arm at the elbow and tensing the muscles of the upper arm. Relax.

5. Tense the muscles of the neck. Push your chin toward your chest, and pulling your head up at the same time, lift your head off the floor. Relax.

6. Tense the muscles of your face. Clamp your jaw tightly shut and pull back on the corners of the mouth. Squint your eyes tightly shut and wrinkle your nose. Raise your eyebrows toward your hairline and wrinkle your forehead. Relax.

7. Tense the muscles of your shoulders, chest, and back. Take a deep breath and hold it. Now pull the shoulders back and together much like the military attention posture. Relax.

8. Tense the muscles of the abdomen. Take a deep breath and bear down with the stomach muscles. Relax.

9. Tense the muscles of the buttocks and right thigh. Press the back of the right knee down into the floor. Relax.

10. Tense the muscles of the right calf and foot. Bend the foot at the ankle and stretch the toes toward the head. Relax.

11. Tense the muscles of the buttocks and left thigh. Press the back of the left knee down into the floor. Relax.

12. Tense the muscles of the left calf and foot. Bend the foot at the ankle and stretch the toes toward the head. Relax.

When you have completed this exercise, take two to three deep breaths and hold each one for a moment, deeply relaxing as you exhale. Enjoy this relaxed state, breathing regularly and slowly to enhance it. Imagery has been found to occur when an individual feels deeply relaxed; if you experience pleasant imagery, allow it to continue and focus on it. When you are ready to end the exercise, slowly count backward from five to one. Move slowly until fully alert. The key to managing your back pain by achieving deep muscular relaxation is to practice every day!

11

ELECTRICAL AND NONSURGICAL PHYSICAL TREATMENTS

Many people mistakenly believe that persistent back pain is, by definition, a surgical problem. Indeed, most patients treated at pain clinics, including the patients I treat at our centers, have undergone one or more unsuccessful major surgeries for pain relief. But by now I hope you are convinced that surgery for back pain is indicated in only a small percentage of cases. If a light burns out in your home you don't automatically consider a costly and extensive electrical rewiring of the house until you have tried a few less costly and simpler remedies first—like changing the light bulb! Unless the evidence for electrical rewiring is clear, changing the bulb or other less intensive efforts are likely to correct the problem. The same is true with a bad back. In the vast majority of cases, the costly and intensive efforts of surgery are simply not required and, in fact, can make your back pain worse!

But if not surgery for back pain relief, then what? Fortunately there is no scarcity of physical treatments for both acute and chronic back pain—ranging from folklore liniments and poultices, to traditional physical therapy modalities, to highly technical and specialized treatment techniques. In fact, let the word out that your back hurts and you will probably learn more about remedies, complete with personal testimonies, than you ever thought possible.

Whether the treatment techniques described in this chapter are truly effective and, if they are, then why they are is a topic of considerable debate. Some of the techniques are understood better than others—and a few are hardly understood at all. We do know that practically any technique will have both positive and negative effects. For example, heat may be useful in decreasing joint pain and stiffness in the patient with arthritis, but may also increase joint swelling. Cold may be used to decrease muscle spasm and pain, but may increase joint pain. How do you decide? Certainly you do not want to aggravate your pain.

The best advice I can offer is to check with your doctor before starting any treatment program. You may not get all of the answers but your doctor is usually in the best position to advise specific treatments. Find a doctor whom you trust. Unfortunately there are a few practitioners who practice what I term "fast food medicine." They have their own theories about the back and will fill you with various "herbs and spices," minerals, and vitamins, and inject you with almost anything short of what is lethal—all under the guise of treatment. Among such injections are sugar, salt water, and phenol (carbolic acid). There is no convincing research evidence documenting the effectiveness of just such injections, but many back pain patients are victimized by the mistaken notion that if a treatment is expensive, it must be good.

Since discussions of every proposed remedy for the back would each represent a literary volume, we will limit this chapter to some of the more traditional and frequently employed electrical and nonsurgical physical treatments for back pain. For a variety of reasons, many sufferers find welcome relief in the treatments. In addition, when compared with surgery and medications, the physical treatment techniques to be described have a low risk factor and are nonaddictive. Some of them may just work for you!

TRANSCUTANEOUS ELECTRICAL NERVE STIMULATION

Electricity's painkilling abilities were well known long before we had any idea what electricity itself was all about, probably as far back as the early Egyptians and the time of Hippocrates. Its first recorded use in that capacity was in 46 A.D. when Scribonius Largus, a Roman physician, used the electric ray or "torpedo fish" in the treatment of headache and gout. Evidently this treatment involved bringing the affected body part into contact with the fish. The electric current would run into the body and relieve the pain, often for hours.

Despite early successes, electrical therapy failed to gain wide support, although occasional reports attesting to its beneficial effects continued into the 1900s. It was not until the 1960s that the analgesic property of electricity was rediscovered. Publication of Melzack and Wall's "gate theory" (Chapter 3) of pain in 1965 renewed interest in the idea of using electrical stimulation in an attempt to control pain.

The initial results were encouraging when small electric-current stimulators were implanted into the spinal column or brain of chronic pain victims. However, this technique carried with it the risk of major surgery and there was no way to predict whether the patient would experience pain relief. What was needed was a safe method of screening for a positive response to electrical stimulation, to determine if surgery for implantation was worth the risk in a particular patient.

Transcutaneous electrical nerve stimulation (TENS) was ideal for this purpose. But during the screening of hundreds of potential candidates for surgical implantation, an interesting phenomenon was discovered. Not only did TENS accurately predict those individuals who might benefit from such surgery, but in many cases the device itself controlled their pain. Enthusiasm for the surgical technique soon decreased as health professionals turned their attention to the harmless electrical box. Scribonius Largus certainly must be laughing from his grave over this discovery by "modern" science.

A TENS unit is basically a battery-powered pulse generator, about the size of a pack of cigarettes, which is usually worn on the belt. A pair of electrodes running from the power unit are attached to the skin directly over the painful area of the body and provide continuous mild electrical stimulation. The intensity of stimulation can be manually controlled by adjusting the dial on the power unit. Most patients familiar with TENS report that it works best if the intensity of stimulation is gradually increased to the point of causing pain, then decreased a bit to provide optimal relief.

The explanation for TENS effectiveness in reducing pain for some individuals remains speculative. Some researchers suggest that TENS interferes with the transmission of pain signals to the brain by forcing the signals to travel large-diameter nerve fibers. Others have proposed a biochemical theory; many believe that TENS induces the release of endorphins (Chapter 3). If you suffer chronic back pain, TENS may help. While it is known that the technique is most effective in acute pain states and that its effectiveness often decreases with time, you will have little to lose in giving TENS a try. Except for excluding individuals who wear cardiac pacemakers, there are no contraindications and practically any physical therapist, technician, or nurse can explain how to use the unit. Discuss the use of TENS with your doctor. Many individuals suffering chronic back pain claim that TENS provides welcome relief.

ELECTRICAL STIMULATION

Like TENS, electrical stimulation has been around for some time. But while some authorities brand the technique quackery, other researchers report the effectiveness of electrical stimulation of tight, spasmed muscles in relieving pain.

As we have discussed in previous chapters, it is rather common that the pain of a chronic back is increased by spasm of spinal muscles. You will recall from the discussion of the "feedback loop of pain" in Chapter 3 that pain often causes muscles to tense and spasm, which causes increased back pain, which causes even more muscular tension and spasm, which causes even more pain, and so on. Electrical stimulation of muscles in spasm has a definite energizing effect that forces the muscles to contract boldly until ultimate muscle fatigue and relaxation occur. When the muscle is finally relaxed, it can be stretched and exercised and this often results in marked pain reduction. Thus the pain relief property of electrical stimulation comes not from the stimulation itself, but rather from the subsequent relaxation of a spasming muscle and ultimate stretching of previously tight, contracted, painful muscles.

Electrical stimulation for back pain is only a mildly uncomfortable procedure. You will usually be asked to lie on your stomach while a therapist or technician administers treatment. The therapist will position one or two wands about the size and shape of a pencil over the area of a painful muscle spasm and send a small electric current into the muscle. You may feel a tingling sensation and also feel the muscle involuntarily contract, but this is only slightly uncomfortable. When the muscle is relaxed, the therapist will usually assist you in stretching and exercising your back and you may well find that you can move about with much less discomfort.

Electrical stimulation is a safe treatment technique that seems to be most effective with acute back pain. Discuss the treatment with your doctor and consider giving it a try. If it helps relieve your back pain, you will probably be given a series of treatments. However, it is most important that you make full use of pain relief. If electrical stimulation works for you, take the opportunity to practice the progressive relaxation exercises (Chapter 10) and stretching and conditioning exercises (Chapter 9) to maximize your long-term back rehabilitation.

THERAPEUTIC HEAT

Similar to the electrical therapies, TENS, and electrical stimulation, the therapeutic use of heat has been recognized for some time, although, perhaps, its use and effectiveness have been underemphasized. Unlike TENS and electrical stimulation, the use of heat to relieve back pain does not always require treatment at a doctor's office or clinic. The local application of heat has been used for the relief of pain since antiquity.

In our age of sophisticated and expensive medical treatments, perhaps the single greatest burden that heat, as an effective treatment technique, has had to bear is its simplicity. Most of us want to be impressed, to try something new, or even "new and improved." We scan magazines to read of new products, new cars, and even new medical treatments. Castigating the tried and true as old-fashioned and outdated, our eyes and attention remain firmly fixed on the future.

Yet heat applied to a painful back can often have a calming, analgesic effect. Muscle spasms and joint stiffness seem to respond particularly well to heat. In addition, heat causes an increase in local blood flow, which is useful in relieving painful inflammatory disorders.

Heat also has side effects and contraindications. Increasing the body temperature may accelerate the destructive process in the joints of individuals with rheumatoid arthritis, although the pain may be temporarily relieved. In addition, heat increases blood flow and vascular dilation to a warmed area, which often worsens an acute inflammatory disorder, as well as increasing swelling after an acute injury.

Several forms of heat are available for back pain. Conductive heat-transfer devices such as electric heating pads or moist heat packs are frequently effective in reducing back discomfort, as is the radiant-heat infrared lamp. Both types of device are useful in heating the skin and tissue just below the skin and both can provide pain relief.

If deeper heating is required, diathermy and ultrasound are available in many doctors' offices and most physical therapy departments. Muscles relatively close to the skin are best treated by diathermy while still deeper structures, such as tendons, ligaments, and very deep muscles, are usually best treated by ultrasound. Both diathermy and ultrasound are sometimes effective in reducing the misery of back pain and, with the exception of some minor muscle twitching, are soothing and pleasant.

Whether infrared lamps, diathermy, and ultrasound provide any pain relief advantages over the old-fashioned remedy of soaking in a hot tub bath is questionable. Many of the back pain victims who come to our centers report little difference in the various heat forms and rely heavily on hot baths for relief. For maximum benefit the bath should last for half an hour. At some point before the 30 minutes are up, the water will begin to feel cooler. Your body will have cooled off a small area of water immediately next to it; if you swish the water around with your hand or move your body about, warmer water will again be positioned against your back.

Soaking in a hot bath twice daily is an inexpensive, soothing, and effective pain relief technique for many people with back pain. It requires no doctors, therapists, prescriptions, or hospital insurance coverage and costs only pennies.

THERAPEUTIC COLD

The local application of cold is another one of grandmother's remedies that has stood the test of time. Like therapeutic heat, cold can decrease muscle spasm and pain and has been used to reduce pain for many years.

The techniques of cold application are not as sophisticated as are those modified versions of the microwave oven we call diathermy and ultrasound. Ice packs, cold wet packs, and various vapocoolant sprays (ethyl chloride, fluorimethane), most frequently seen sprayed on injured baseball and football players, are the methods generally used to administer cold. However, at our centers we have a different way of using cold to relieve chronic back pain. We call the technique "ice massage."

The process is relatively simple and you or a family member can serve as therapist. Fill a paper cup with water and drop a wooden ice cream stick into the cup. Put the cup in your freezer and wait for the water to harden into ice. Remove the cup and tear away the paper covering and you have a cake of ice on a stick, like a popsicle.

Next, remove your shirt and have someone place the cake of ice directly on your painful back. To avoid freezing and damaging the skin, do not leave the ice on one part of your back for more than a second or two. Press the ice onto the back while moving the cake in either a circular or back-and-forth motion.

Patients treated at our centers describe the stages of ice massage as four separate sensations in a five- to ten-minute period. An initial cold feeling is followed by one of burning, then a mild aching, then numbness, at which point the massage is stopped. If you are hypersensitive to cold, this treatment is not recommended.

Many of our patients report initial relief for only 15 to 20 minutes, but with continued treatment, pain relief can sometimes be increased to three or four hours at a time. In addition, an ice massage before bed followed by practice in progressive relaxation (Chapter 10) can assist chronic back pain victims in getting to sleep without drugs.

With back pain second only to headaches as a chronic health problem, do not be fooled into thinking that relief must be costly and complicated. For the motivated victim of chronic back pain, the refrigerator can be an extension of your medicine chest, even if the only things in it are ice cubes!

NERVE BLOCKS

If your doctor believes that all or part of your pain has resulted from an injured or damaged nerve, he or she may recommend blocking the nerve in order to interrupt the message of pain carried by the nerve to the brain. "Nerve blocks" are various techniques that involve placing a small-caliber needle through the skin and advancing it to the area of the nerve suspected of contributing to or causing pain. A local anesthetic or alcohol mixture is injected through the needle for the purpose of diagnosis and/or temporary pain relief.

Unfortunately nerve blocks are not always effective. When they do "take," the relief is usually only temporary (four to eight hours). Some doctors believe that repeated blocks over a period of weeks can result in prolonged relief from pain, but others question the long-term effectiveness of blocks. Nevertheless nerve blocks are relatively harmless techniques that have been used for years in selected surgical and obstetrical cases. Besides the pin prick produced by the needle as it punctures the skin, you may expect an occasional muscle twitch or "electricity" feeling in the area of the body affected by the nerve.

Soon after the procedure you may experience dizziness, some shaking and sweating, occasional minor headache, and soreness in the area where the needle was introduced. Some consequences of nerve blocking may be caused by anxiety and these fade away as the nerve block therapy proceeds.

Nerve blocks may also cause feelings of warmness, and numbness and weakness in the limbs, depending on the bodily region that has been blocked. If the nerve block involves the face and neck, you may experience eyelid droop and hoarseness. These problems are transitory, and recovery can be expected within ten to 12 hours following the procedure.

Other possible, but improbable, complications include various disturbances in vital organ functions and biorhythms, such as changes in breathing, blood pressure, and states of awareness. Such complications generally follow soon after the injection of the analgesic drug. Serious side effects of nerve blocks very rarely are seen.

If you complain of pain long enough, you will surely find someone anxious to perform a nerve block or series of blocks despite the fact that with chronic back pain this treatment is seldom effective. Nerve blocks may have the advantages of being nonaddictive, repeatable, less risky than surgery, and as not requiring hospitalization, but the same can be said for hundreds of other noneffective treatments for chronic pain.

ACUPUNCTURE

A 56-year-old man slowly limps across the parking lot, holding his back as he makes his way into the doctor's office. An hour later, after acupuncture treatment, he retraces his steps with no limp or other sign of back pain. A 30-year-old female watches while the surgeon cuts away a large bunion from her foot. The operation completed, he applies the cast as she calmly chats and sips milk. A few minutes later, the surgeon removes an array of stainless steel needles from the patient's upper arm, nose, and ears, the only anesthetic she requested for the surgery.

Over a decade ago, *New York Times* columnist James Reston wrote glowingly of how acupuncture relieved pressure and distension after his appendectomy in Peking. That article, combined with President Nixon's policy of recognizing China, provided Americans with a "new" national fascination—acupuncture! Soon T-shirts and bumper stickers were seen proclaiming the virtues of acupuncture and acupuncturists were in business across the nation. Newspaper and magazine articles heralded acupuncture as a "new medical miracle" and thousands of pain sufferers journeyed to acupuncture centers for relief and cure.

The acupuncture fad had disastrous results. Acupuncture treatment was applied indiscriminately by poorly trained practitioners who were neither licensed nor required to demonstrate any degree of clinical competency. Although there were some serious and legitimate practitioners, most adhered to the "strike while the iron is hot" philosophy of business. Acupuncture did wonders to increase the bank accounts of corrupt practitioners but little or nothing to relieve the suffering of pain. In time acupuncture lost favor with many enthusiasts and patients desperate for pain relief.

Is there a place for acupuncture in relieving pain? What are patients and doctors to make of this ancient medical art imported from the Orient? Does it work? Is it safe? Can it provide you relief from back pain?

Perhaps the best way to answer these questions is to realize that acupuncture is not a "medical miracle," nor is it a new treatment. Insertion of needles into the skin at strategic points of the body to treat disease and pain goes back nearly 5000 years in China, and versions of the art were also practiced by the ancient Egyptians and others. The early Chinese believed acupuncture would supply an almost certain way of maintaining equilibrium of the body, which was seen as a sort of energy field, with lines of force called currents running exact routes along a network of meridians. Along the network, at specific points, were several hundred centers that controlled the energy field—the acupuncture points.

Illness and pain occurred when a person's energy became unbalanced and there was too much energy in one part of the body, too little in another. What was needed to overcome pain and restore balance, or so it was thought, was to have an acupuncturist insert needles into these crucial points and twirl them rapidly, so that the oversupply of energy from one area would be shunted to the region of undersupply. The fact that patients often improved or lost their pain was good enough evidence for its practitioners. Even so, it was not until 1958, after years of medical and political debate, that China adopted acupuncture as an anesthetic for major operations, including brain and lung surgery. Now acupuncture is used to deaden pain in about 20 percent of all surgery in China, although tranquilizers may be given before surgery to relax the patient.

Both Chinese and American medical researchers are at a loss to explain the effectiveness of acupuncture. Some equate it with the placebo response and relate it to suggestibility, concentration, distraction, expectancy, and other psychological phenomena. Other scientists believe that acupuncture stimulates certain nerve pathways to send messages to the brain to counteract pain messages.

Recently an important clue to the puzzle of how acupuncture works was discovered by researchers who detected in patients treated with acupuncture the increased presence of endorphins. You will recall from Chapter 3 that endorphins are morphinelike biochemical substances that act as the body's own painkillers. Why insertion of needles into the body encourages the supply of endorphins is unclear, but the discovery of some relationship between acupuncture and endorphins is considered a major breakthrough in better understanding this ancient therapy.

Can acupuncture help relieve your pain? In my experience the answer is perhaps, but not likely. Because of this statement, I'm sure to receive letters of disagreement from former pain patients who can provide detailed case histories of their once painful backs as evidence that acupuncture is an effective treatment technique that worked when nothing else did. To these fortunate individuals, I offer my apologies, but also maintain that practically any "treatment," from sprinkling salt to mystical chanting, will be effective in highly isolated and individual situations. The laws of statistical probability include a small margin of error, and it is with this in mind that I report that research has failed to identify acupuncture as an effective treatment technique for back pain.

However, if your back pain has not responded to other types of treatment and you have a desire to investigate acupuncture further, by all means do so. The technique is relatively safe and painless when practiced by a competent practitioner. The risk of acupuncture is not so much that a needle will be inserted improperly, but that the practitioner, failing to recognize a serious underlying disease, may cause you to delay going for conventional medical treatment.

Most acupuncture centers charge from $40 to $75 per treatment and the average course of treatment for back pain runs from eight to 12 sessions.

ACCUPRESSURE

Accupressure is very much like acupuncture except for two distinguishing characteristics: (1) needles that puncture the skin are not used, and (2) rather than concentrating on ancient and well-known acupuncture points, accupressure involves identifying "trigger points" that may or may not correspond to traditional acupuncture points. In other words, accupressure involves searching the body for small sensitive areas, which, when pressured, cause pain in another part of the body. For victims of low back pain, trigger points may be located in various parts of the body, including the upper back, shoulder, and legs (Figure 11-1). Once trigger points are identified, they can be broken up by pressing a blunt object, such as the fingertip or knuckle, into the trigger area and the spasm may dissolve.

The term "trigger" is descriptive since stimulation of the unduly sensitive small muscle areas, like pulling the trigger on a gun, can produce effects in other parts of the body, or target areas. When stimulation of one body part creates pain in a different part of the body, the discomfort is called *referred* pain. Referred pain may be only dull and aching, but it can also be severe. For example, if the back as a target area is pressed, there may be only a slight increase in discomfort. But if the same amount of pressure is applied to a trigger point, the pain increase in the target area (back) is sharp.

Considerable mystery surrounds the trigger point phenomenon. How does a trigger point arise? At some time virtually all of us have experienced the cramping of a calf muscle in a leg as millions of muscle fibers suddenly contract to knot the muscle. There is one theory that a trigger point may develop when, for some reason, perhaps under the stress of severe spasm, just a few thousand fibers tighten and form a localized knot that may persist even after the spasm disappears.

Whatever the mechanism of formation, when a trigger point is present and causing pain, treatment of that point may bring dramatic relief. Within minutes pain that has persisted for months may disappear completely, and sometimes permanently.

If the phenomenon of accupressure treatment interests you, take a few moments to study Figure 11-1 before searching your body for

ACUPRESSURE TRIGGER POINTS

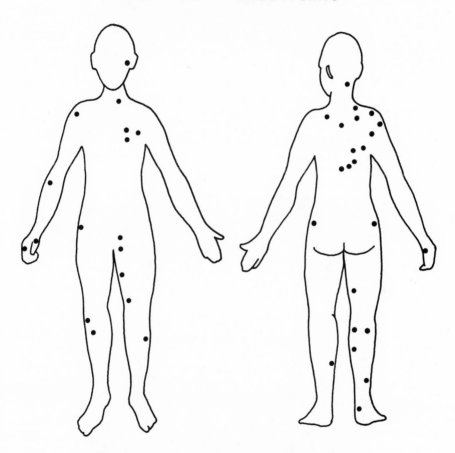

Figure 11-1—"Trigger points" can sometimes be located in various parts of the body. Stimulation of the point may "trigger" pain in a different body part, including the lower back.

trigger points. Of course, not every victim of chronic back pain will have trigger points so do not be concerned if you cannot locate these small sensitive nodules. If you do locate one or more trigger points, you may wish to identify them to your doctor, or even attempt to dissolve the spasm yourself. This can sometimes be done by pressing a knuckle into the trigger area and rotating it in a circular fashion. If your location is a true trigger point, pressing the area will probably cause increased pain in the target area of your back until the point is dissolved and your pain eases. Accupressure trigger point therapy may be a "long-shot" treatment for your back pain, but there are pain victims who claim it works.

12

BIOFEEDBACK TRAINING

In the late 1960s and early 1970s, we were bombarded with media claims of a new scientific breakthrough that would revolutionize health care. From the common cold to leukemia, a wide variety of human illnesses were reported to respond to the new mind-control technique of biofeedback. I recall standing casually in a supermarket line some years ago and thumbing through a new biofeedback book on sale entitled *Your Mind Can Stop the Common Cold*. Other early claims for biofeedback included:

- An extraordinary technique that allows you to control the state of your health, happiness, and well-being through the power of your mind.
- A spectacular scientific theory that has become fact in hospitals and laboratories across the country.
- A revolutionary method of getting quickly in touch with the inner self.
- Something yogis and Zen masters have been doing for centuries to achieve inner peace and joy.
- A visionary technology that places the power for change and control in the hands of individuals and allows them to control their own destinies.

Biofeedback was initially offered as a miracle treatment for practically every medical disorder that had proved resistant to conventional methods of treatment. Unfortunately the early claims made for biofeedback were grossly exaggerated. Today we know that it is not a miracle treatment nor has it revolutionized health care. We also know that biofeedback will not cure the common cold, cancer, leukemia, heart disease, or kidney disease. Biofeedback is simply a treatment technique, albeit a proven, effective treatment technique in carefully selected patients suffering a limited number of medical problems that have not responded well to traditional medical practices. It is just one of many treatment techniques available for use by doctors to treat such stubborn problems as chronic anxiety, tension headaches and migraine headaches, and chronic pain. Still research continues to explore the possibility that one day individuals may be able to exert a degree of control over physiological systems involved in many serious medical disorders that continue to defy medical science.

The historical roots of biofeedback can be traced back to the fascination of scientists and lay people alike with Far Eastern yogis who reportedly can walk on hot coals without being burned, submerge themselves in water for prolonged periods without oxygen, and recline on beds of sharp nails without injury. While many individuals suspect deceit and trickery in such demonstrations, a small number of scientists became interested in exploring the ability to exert mental control over physiological processes long thought to be involuntary in nature.

Scientists interested in rigorously testing such feats organized to monitor and analyze the physiological changes that take place in these practitioners. A classic investigation of yogic self-control of the body was conducted by Marion A. Wenger in 1961 (with B. K. Bagchi, "Studies of Autonomic Functions in Practitioners of Yoga in India," *Behavioral Science*, 1961). Nearly a decade later, the Menninger Foundation in Topeka, Kans., invited an Indian yogi, H. H. Swami Rama, to participate in a project exploring voluntary control of internal states. During the swami's first physicological recording session, he demonstrated an ability to increase the temperature of the left side of one hand several degrees higher than that of the right side of the same hand. Later in this session, the swami "stopped" his heart for 17 seconds. Actually, though the EKG reading of his heartbeat appeared perfectly flat, the swami in fact *increased* his heart rate to over 300 beats per minute, about three times normal. He can maintain this increased heart rate up to three minutes at a time.

Additional and highly influential support for the belief in the ability to control autonomic or involuntary body responses appeared in 1969 in a series of papers by Dr. Neil Miller and his associates at Rockefeller University. Dr. Miller, a psychologist, demonstrated in a series of investigations that rats could be trained to modify their heart rate, blood pressure, urine formation, intestinal contractions, and other responses of the autonomic nervous system that were previously thought to be involuntary.

The general technique used in these studies involved the rats receiving a very pleasant electrical stimulation to the brain as a reinforcer or reward for autonomic nervous system changes in the required direction. In other words, if the researcher wanted the rat to decrease its heart rate, a reward was given each time the heart rate slowed, no matter how gradual the decrease. This technique is termed *shaping* and soon the rats became more proficient at decreasing their heart rate. Most of the rats were temporarily paralyzed with the drug curare prior to each learning trial in order to rule out the possibility that the autonomic changes were due simply to changes in respiration, muscle activity, or both. The results of experimentation were surprising. Not only were large changes in autonomic system responses produced, but the changes were often quite specific. For example, in one experiment rats were trained to increase the blood flow to one ear while maintaining the natural flow of blood to the other! Needless to say, this caught the eye and imagination of researchers worldwide and scientists were quick to recognize the potential of this work for teaching patients with physiological disorders to exert some voluntary degree of control over the medical problem.

After over two decades of research, there are now volumes of controlled scientific investigations documenting the clinical effectiveness of biofeedback training. Such research has altered the traditional view of the nervous system—one that most of us were probably taught in basic biology classes in school—that many of the body's functions are involuntary and virtually automatic. Of course, it is as true as it ever was that our hearts beat whether we will them to or not, our lungs fill and empty whether we are awake or asleep, and our digestive processes operate more or less independently of the conscious attention we may pay them. But it was assumed for years that the independent operation of these functions meant that there was no way for us to exert conscious control over them, which is not the case. It is now clear that we can influence these processes and others, sometimes profoundly, and that electronic biofeedback instruments can expand and refine our ability to do so. The ability to control one's physiology varies among individuals. Some people learn it quickly, others only with difficulty or not at all; and for many body processes, we have not yet been able to show that conscious effort—even with electronic assistance—can produce meaningful levels of change. But we have a much more active role to play in the way our bodies function than was once thought possible. And what was once a counterculture fad of achieving inner peace through alpha-wave feedback is today routinely performed by doctors in treating a variety of human medical disorders, including back pain.

WHAT IS BIOFEEDBACK?

To understand biofeedback and how it may work for you, a distinction must first be drawn between biofeedback and biofeedback training. Biofeedback may be defined as the use of monitoring instruments to record and display physiological activity within the body. The purpose of this procedure is to make this information available to the individual. Using this definition, a number of rather common medical instruments qualify as biofeedback, including a thermometer, stethoscope, and even the bathroom scales. Biofeedback can therefore be thought of as a shorthand expression to describe the process of "feeding back" biological information to the individual generating the information.

If an individual takes internal biological activity that is measured in some way and continuously "fed back", and attempts to use the information to guide trial-and-error efforts to modify the targeted biological activity, biofeedback training is being used. To employ an elementary example, take an ordinary oral thermometer and tape the thermometer bulb to the fatty pad of the tip of the middle finger. Make sure there is good contact between the bulb and fingertip, but be careful not to restrict the circulation. A thermometer, of course, measures body temperature and feeds the information back to the interested individual, and so qualifies under our basic definition of biofeedback. However, now we want to go a step further and use the thermometer to engage in biofeedback training. After five minutes or so of quietly sitting with the eyes closed, note the temperature of the finger. Then, while still in position, try to relax and slowly repeat several autosuggestions to yourself, such as, "I am feeling warm and relaxed," "My hands feel warm like they were in a pan of very warm water." Repeat the suggestions slowly, allowing them to take effect, and relax. Every five minutes or so, take note of the finger temperature. Most individuals will show a rise in finger temperature after ten to 20 minutes, some increasing their finger temperature four to five, or even ten, degrees, some only one or two degrees. A few people will not increase finger temperature, and may even decrease the temperature, but with practice, everyone can learn this very basic biofeedback training technique.

This elementary demonstration includes all of the basic components of biofeedback and biofeedback training. First, there is monitoring of a physiological activity within the body, the thermometer recording body temperature. Second, the physiological activity is fed back and made available. Third, there is an implicit intention to alter the targeted physiological activity, in this case, to increase finger temperature. Fourth, trial-and-error learning is required to master physiological control. Finally, there is an as-yet-indescribable mental mechanism that exerts an effect on the targeted physicological activity. The result is voluntary control over an internal physiological activity considered for years to be beyond our control. One research scientist further explains biofeedback as follows:

The general term biofeedback was coined by the mathematician Norbert Weiner and concisely defined by him as "a method of controlling a system by reinserting into it the results of its past performance." Biofeedback, then, is a special case of this, where the system is a biological system and where the feedback is artificial, mediated by man-made detection, amplification, and display instruments, rather than being present as an inborn feedback loop inherent within the biologic system. Biologically, then, one should not be so surprised at the efficacy of biofeedback, since every animal is a self-regulated system owing its existence, its stability and most of its behavior to feedback controls. Every infant, for example, learns hand–eye coordination (and even the whole concept of space and distance) by means of visual proprioceptive feedback. By repeated trial-and-error learning, through feedback, eventually the infant comes to be able to control his arms and hand muscles quite precisely, and to reach accurately toward where things are in space, choosing the right direction, distance, angle of approach, and width of grasp on the basis of prior feedback-gained experience. In a way, then, the real surprising thing is not that biofeedback should work at all, but that it was not experimentally looked for and so discovered earlier than it was. (Yemm, R., *Archives of Oral Biology*, 1969, 14:874.)

BIOFEEDBACK TRAINING: TECHNIQUE

There are two basic facts that must be recognized before fully understanding biofeedback and how biofeedback training may help you better control pain or other health problems. First, biomedical authority and psychophysiology for years have taught the doctrine that neither humans nor animals could control those internal physiological activities of the body's vital functions. These functions are regulated by involuntary automatic control systems and by reflexes, long considered to be beyond the control of the mind. There was, and still is to a few scientists, no such thing as the mind, only brain, and certainly no such thing as mind over matter. Mind was only an illusion about the mysteries of the brain. However, a large number of controlled scientific investigations documenting the effectiveness of biofeedback training are now gradually eliminating this outdated mode of thought.

Second, it should be fully recognized that biofeedback training drastically changes the traditional doctor–patient relationship. Most health care is based on an active–passive model, the doctor actively administering health care to the passive recipient patient. Biofeedback training is different. Biofeedback training requires that the patient assume responsibility for learning the techniques required to alter targeted physiological activity and thereby achieving the desired control over an identified medical disorder. The doctor functions more as a "coach" or "educator" in assisting the patient to learn control of internal activity. The biofeedback patient must recognize this modification of tradition and be willing to assume responsibility for the success of biofeedback training. With this in mind, let us look at how biofeedback training is conducted.

Probably the most effective use of biofeedback in the treatment of chronic pain has focused on learning voluntary control of targeted muscle groups in the body. Since much of the discomfort of back pain is caused by muscular spasm in various areas of the spine, this is particularly relevant to individuals suffering back pain. The term given to this type of biofeedback training is electromyographic feedback, more commonly referred to as EMG biofeedback. EMG is but one of several types of biofeedback and involves measuring and recording the electrical activity of targeted muscles and feeding back this information to the patient, who uses the information, along with instructions from the doctor, to learn better control of "tight" or "tense" muscles. We know that back pain and spasm are usually synonymous with muscle tension throughout the body. In fact, because of the body's natural homeostatic adaption, many victims of chronic back pain, including extremely tense and rigid muscles, do not recognize their level of tension and the state of their musculature.

Should you and your doctor decide that biofeedback training is indicated in an effort to manage your back discomfort better, you will learn that biofeedback involves several phases. While different doctors vary in their personal approach, the following protocol should give you some idea of what to expect.

The first phase of biofeedback training is the recording of muscle activity in order to establish a baseline measure of your muscle tension. You will likely be asked to sit in a comfortable chair, usually in a dimly lit, sound-resistant room. Near you will be the biofeedback equipment, which may remind you of a collection of stereo components complete with meters, calibration dials, and flashing lights. Your doctor will orient you to the equipment and will attach two or more small electrodes to the skin directly over a selected muscle group in your body. With individuals suffering chronic back pain, the upper trapezius (shoulder and neck muscles) and paraspinal muscles (muscles adjacent to either side of the spine) are two favorite targets for treatment since most research indicates that the upper trapezius muscles provide the best general assessment of overall body tension (Figure 12-1) and the paraspinal muscles fre-

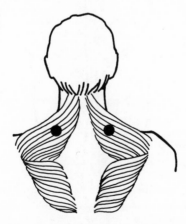

Figure 12-1—Measurement of "muscle tension" in the trapezius muscles is often considered the best indicator of overall body tension.

quently spasm, causing increased back discomfort (Figure 12-2).

Before the electrodes are applied with adhesive collars or an elastic band, the skin will be thoroughly cleaned with alcohol or acetate to facilitate optimal contact between the skin and electrodes. You will next be asked to relax while a resting level or baseline measure of the electrical activity of the muscles is recorded. This will indicate the state and degree of muscle tension or relaxation. The baseline measure is considered a starting point for treatment. Over the next several sessions, you will gradually learn to reduce the tension in the muscles so that your baseline measure after six to 12 training sessions is greatly reduced compared with the initial baseline recording.

Once a baseline has been established, it is time to begin biofeedback training. You will recall from the earlier discussion of the laboratory rats taught to control internal physiological activities that

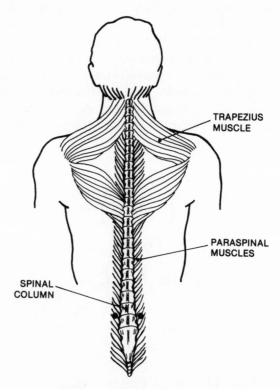

Figure 12-2—Spasming and tension of the paraspinal muscles can increase back pain.

the basis of biofeedback is a process known as shaping. Shaping is a basic learning technique whereby progress toward an identified goal is accomplished through small, incremental steps. One step must be successfully mastered before proceeding to the next. Since a reduction in muscle tension is the goal of chronic back pain patients, your doctor will set a threshold so that a soft tone continuously sounds. Successful muscle relaxation will terminate the tone, thereby signaling that you have successfully decreased your muscle tension. A new, slightly more difficult threshold is then set, which you will work to terminate by further relaxing your muscles. The pitch of the tone keeps you constantly informed of your muscle tension level. An increase in muscle tension results in an immediate higher pitched tone and a decrease in muscle tension results in a lower pitched tone. Again, the object is to terminate the tone by decreasing the tension in your muscles and learn to control your muscles and pain. Step-by-step levels of muscle tension are gradually reduced through shaping until you arrive at a level where the muscles are no longer tense and your discomfort is decreased. The more you practice the biofeedback technique, the easier relaxing your muscles becomes.

After you begin to demonstrate moderate control of the muscle tension, your doctor or therapist may introduce a voluntary control phase to the training protocol. During the voluntary control phase, you will not be given feedback. Rather, your doctor or therapist monitors your progress while you exert passive voluntary control of the targeted physiological process. Voluntary control phases instituted in the overall training protocol prohibit excessive dependence on continuous feedback to control muscle tension and help generalize your ability to control the muscular tension outside of the doctor's office. When you are able to control your muscle tension during the voluntary control phase, your doctor may ask you to begin practicing the control technique at home between training sessions.

If you asked successful biofeedback patients how they voluntarily exercise control over biological processes long thought to be beyond our control, most would probably say that they were not sure. Some patients report concentrating on peaceful thoughts while others say they imagine floating on a cloud. A few even report concentrating on sexual fantasies. Regardless of what specific imagery is used, the majority of biofeedback patients report that successful control is something of a "knack" or "sense," much like the sense of knowing the position of your arm even when your eyes are closed. They further report that during early training, control over internal physiological activity requires intense concentration and effort, but over time becomes a technique that requires very little conscious effort.

UPPER BACK, NECK, AND HEAD PAIN

When chronic pain concentrates in the area of the upper back, neck, and head, the trapezius muscles (Figure 12-1) are generally found to be in spasm and contributing to the discomfort. Biofeedback training for upper back, neck, and head pain is based on the following premise: If muscular tension in the neck, shoulders, and head can be decreased, or prevented before it begins, and can be maintained at reduced levels, the frequency and intensity of pain can be reduced, or even eliminated. EMG biofeedback is again generally considered to be the most effective type of biofeedback training. Electrodes are usually attached to the neck or shoulders (trapezius muscles), depending on which area is identified as having the greatest level of muscular tension and which part of the back and neck is identified as the location of the pain. EMG biofeedback training is then performed as previously described until the individual learns voluntarily to control the level of muscle activity and to reduce or eliminate the pain. As with biofeedback treatment of most medical or psychological disorders, a multimodal treatment program combining biofeedback training with other treatment techniques described in this book seems to facilitate long-term success.

LOW BACK PAIN

Biofeedback training for chronic low back pain is one of the newest and least documented uses of biofeedback training. Theoretically the effectiveness of treatment is based on the "feedback loop of pain" (Figure 3-1). According to the feedback loop of pain, the perception of pain causes increased muscle tension throughout the body. If you have ever closed an automobile door on your finger or dropped a heavy object on your foot, you are aware that the entire body reacts to the onset of pain with a dramatic surge of energy as the muscles spring to attention and prepare for some action to escape the pain. If the pain subsides in a short time, the muscles will gradually relax and the physiology of the body returns to normal. However, if the pain does not subside, as is the case with chronic back pain, the muscles remain tense and rigid indefinitely. We know that muscles that are tense and rigid for prolonged periods will themselves become painful. You can demonstrate this by making a tight fist and holding the muscle tension in your hand. After a few minutes, the hand will become so painful you will be forced to release the tension and relax the muscles. Chronic low back pain victims often suffer two problems—the initial pain from whatever tissue damage occurred in the back and secondary pain that results from tense and rigid muscles. To make matters worse, the two sources of pain combine to form a feedback loop, the initial pain causing muscle tension that creates more pain, which causes even more muscle tension, and so on.

Most doctors believe that the value of EMG biofeedback in the treatment of low back pain is general muscle relaxation, which breaks the feedback loop of pain. Electrodes are attached to the area of the lower back and feedback of muscle activity is provided for the patient who practices techniques to lower muscular tension. Research continues to define the ultimate ability of biofeedback training in chronic low back pain.

OTHER TYPES OF BIOFEEDBACK

In addition to electromyographic, or EMG, biofeedback, several other types of biofeedback are currently employed in the treatment of human illnesses. While EMG is the biofeedback treatment of choice with disorders such as muscular tension, insomnia, anxiety, tension headaches, asthma, hypertension, and menstrual distress, galvanic skin response and temperature training have also proved effective as treatment techniques in carefully selected health problems.

Galvanic Skin Response

Galvanic skin response (GSR) biofeedback instruments measure skin conductivity or electrical resistance, which is considered a measurement of emotional autonomic nervous system arousal. Historically this process has been popularized for its use in lie detectors. The theoretical explanation of lie detectors is based partly on scientific research and partly on the general assumption that telling a lie creates in humans a state of increased autonomic nervous system activity and general emotional arousal. This response results in a minute increase in the activity of the sweat glands that alters the conductivity and electrical resistance of the skin and is detected by small GSR electrodes.

In biofeedback training a state of increased autonomic nervous system activity and general emotional arousal is considered by many scientists to be very similar to that psychophysiologic state we generally term "anxiety" or "nervousness." As such GSR biofeedback is frequently employed in the treatment of hyperhydrosis (excessive sweating), which accompanies anxiety states in some people. In addition, GSR biofeedback training is occasionally used in the treatment of generalized anxiety, although most research favors EMG biofeedback training as more clinically effective for the treatment of anxiety and tension.

Temperature Training

Temperature training monitors minute fluctuations in body temperature, which are thought to be a measure of autonomic nervous system activity. This is measured by using hand or finger temperature. A small sensor is usually attached to the middle or little finger and temperature charges are monitored and transmitted to a biofeedback integrator unit for amplification and visual and/or audio display. Since body temperature is, in part, a function of the volume of blood flow in the body, temperature biofeedback training is often quite successfully employed in the treatment of migraine headaches and vascular problems associated with cold hands and feet, such as Raynaud's disease. It is believed that training an individual to raise the temperature of the hands, through trial-and-error continuous feedback of body temperature, produces an antistress or relaxation response. When the autonomic nervous system is relaxed, headaches usually subside or can be prevented from occurring and cold hands and feet resulting from arterial constriction can often be warmed. In clinical practice temperature and EMG biofeedback training are frequently used simultaneously to monitor and feed back tension and anxiety in both the autonomic and the voluntary nervous system.

13

DIET, NUTRITION, AND SLEEP

If I told you that over 50 percent of all men and women in this country need to lose weight, would you believe me? What if I said 60 percent? According to statistics, over 65 *percent* of all adults in the United States need to lose weight, and the numbers are growing every year. Furthermore, it is a safe bet that even those individuals who maintain proper body weight do not consistently eat the right foods and know little about how various foods influence our health. What a pity that so few realize the role that nutrition plays in the maintenance and rebuilding of our health and strength, including the health of our backs. It is frightening to observe what foods many people consume on the assumption that they provide the nourishment we need—white flour and white sugar products; refined and processed cereals; all types of canned foods, pickled, preserved, and processed meats. Practically every food brought into the American home from the conventional food store is tampered with in one way or another and so falls far short of providing the nourishment we need for the building, or rebuilding, of a healthy, vigorous back and body.

And how about sleep? How many of us have sleeping problems? According to research conducted at our centers, over 90 percent of back pain victims have problems falling asleep, staying asleep for more than a few hours, or both.

Diet, nutrition, and sleep are three critical factors that greatly influence the health of our backs, as well as our overall health and well-being. Yet how many of us take the initiative to control our weight? Consider the following myths:

1. Body weight has little to do with back pain.
2. Diet pills and fad diets are not harmful or they would not be so readily available.
3. Food has little to do with the way we feel.
4. Food has little to do with our mood and optimism.
5. Sleep is a natural state beyond any control on our part.
6. Sleeping pills are not harmful or doctors would not prescribe them.

If you suffer back pain and are overweight, do not eat the proper foods, and also have sleep problems, you owe it to yourself to modify your life-style. This chapter will tell you how. But if you have really "bought in" to the six myths outlined, you have a decision to make. You can skip this section and move on to Chapter 14, put this book down and refuse to read the remainder, or carefully read this chapter and give me a chance to change your mind. The decision is yours. I hope you decide on the last.

DIET

Americans hunger for diets. The average American goes on and off 1.4 diets per year. In the search for slimness, dieters drink gallons of water, diet colas, and grapefruit juice; munch on rice, carrots, and celery; and satiate themselves with yogurt and cottage cheese. The results of our obsession with diets can have both positive and negative effects. For example, the rush to slimness often has physical costs. Diets can cause headaches, dizziness, diarrhea, fatigue, indigestion, skin problems, and constipation. There are also psychological costs. Dieters often suffer from irritability and depression. They sacrifice, agonize, and lose sleep, but they seldom stay thin. The problem is that effective and permanent weight control requires concentrating just as much on behavior as on food.

For everyone, including those who say, "I was meant to be fat," or "Obesity runs in my family," or "I have a hormone problem," being overweight means consuming more calories than the body uses. Adults usually require around 2200 calories for good health. How many calories a person needs above or under that level depends upon his or her metabolic rate, amount of activity, and present weight.

Calories that are not needed to maintain our body functioning or to serve as fuel to move us about are converted into fat. The fat-

TABLE 13-1
APPROXIMATE CALORIE EXPENDITURE

Body weight is, in part, a function of caloric intake versus caloric expenditure.

Activity	Calories/Hour
Lying down/sleeping	80
Sitting	100
Driving a car	120
Standing	140
Housework	180
Walking, 2½ mph	210
Bicycling, 5½ mph	210
Gardening	220
Golf, lawn mowing	250
Bowling	270
Walking, 3¾ mph	300
Swimming, ¼ mph	300
Square dancing	350
Volley ball, rollerskating	350
Wood chopping, sawing	400
Tennis	420
Skiing, 10 mph	600
Squash, handball	600
Bicycling, 13 mph	660
Running, 10 mph	900

conversion formula varies from person to person, but the average is one pound of fat for every 3,500 excess calories. Consider this: Consume a little over 100 extra calories per day—a handful of peanuts, a glass of beer, or even a large apple—and in one month you are one pound heavier! Eat peanuts while you drink the beer and you are two pounds heavier. In a year it is possible to go from thin to fat without ever being a pig!

Occasional binges add up the same way. A person may eat sensibly all week, but extra servings of cake on the weekends will mean that extra pounds will slowly appear. In addition, most people become less active as they grow older, and this has the same result as eating more. A person suddenly sidelined with a back injury who continues eating the same amount of food will gain weight. In fact, the back pain patients we see at our centers have averaged a gain of 21 pounds since the onset of back pain!

Big Bellies and Bad Backs

Two questions I am asked every day are: (1) I was overweight before my back started hurting, so what has weight to do with my back pain? (2) It's not my stomach that hurts, it's my back. What does my weight have to do with my back hurting?

The answer is this: Extra pounds can both *cause* back trouble and complicate *recovery* from back pain. This is not to say that every low back problem is caused by excessive weight (although many are), nor am I saying that every overweight person can expect to experience the onset of back discomfort. The causes and cures of back pain are seldom that simple.

But of all the muscles that support the low back, the abdominal muscles are the most neglected, and among the most important. The weak abdominal muscles of a protruding tummy or after a pregnancy do not "pull their load" with the other back supporting muscles and backache can result. Figure 13-1 shows the increased pressure on the lower back when gravity works its natural force on a potbelly. As more weight accumulates in the stomach, the natural center of gravity is disrupted and the body will fall forward unless the back works extra duty to hold us upright. The result is extra work for an already bad back and increased back pain. I sometimes tell my patients that to expect a bad back to carry excessive weight is similar to expecting a small Volkswagon engine to pull the weight of a Cadillac or other large automobile. Losing excess pounds can remove a sizable load, and while you may not enjoy total pain relief, you can expect reduced pain and better health.

Preparing to Diet

Before jumping into some bizarre fad diet advertised to help you "lose five pounds a day," let us discuss proper and scientific dieting. For your health's sake, you want to lose weight gradually, but regularly, and, most important, keep it off. Don't attempt to save your back by losing your health through fasting or improper weight loss. Remember that proper weight control depends just as much on changing your behavior as changing what and how much you eat. Be sensible. Have a weight loss "game plan" based on a thorough analysis of your eating habits.

The first step is to identify the problem. If you are overweight,

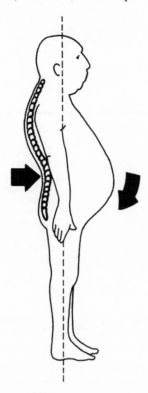

Figure 13-1—The gravitational pull of a protruded abdomen can increase the work demands of the lower back and cause increased pain.

you are doing something wrong and the first step is to find out what. Perhaps you are eating too much, eating the wrong kinds of foods, or exercising too little. The more overweight you are, the more likely it is that you are having problems with all three areas.

The second step is to pay close attention to *what* you eat, *how much* you eat, and *when* you eat. How often do we see the person who eats only three moderate and balanced meals each day but supplements these diet meals with a midmorning donut, an afternoon piece of candy, and a midnight snack?

The third step is to consider how best to solve the problems identified in steps one and two. Perhaps you need to change the types of foods you eat, exercise more, change the times that you eat, eliminate between-meal snacks, or reduce your food intake. Be honest with yourself.

TABLE 13-2
EATING HABITS

Like most other human behaviors,
eating may be influenced by any number of good
and bad habits.

Bad	Good
1. Taking second helpings	Eating only amount allowed
2. Eating between meals	Eating only at appointed time and place
3. Gulping down food	Eating slowly, chewing thoroughly
4. Eating more when you feel full	Stopping when you feel satisfied
5. Eating while watching TV	Selecting foods from the free list
6. Nibbling	Choosing low-calorie foods, if necessary
7. Tasting unnecessarily	Chewing sugar-free gum or mints
8. Finishing leftovers	Brushing teeth to avoid this
9. Eating standing up	Sitting down, relaxing
10. Having to eat alone	Serving in a plate, putting leftovers away, then sitting in a relaxed pleasant atmosphere
11. Irregular eating pattern	Eating three meals per day at scheduled times
12. Eating when tense, upset	Taking a walk first
13. Eating when you need to make a decision	Taking a walk, thinking things out first
14. Eating when lonely	Calling a friend, window shopping
15. Being depressed or bored	Developing a hobby, joining a club
16. Grieving	Visiting someone, talking
17. Being tired	Sleeping regularly, resting first, or exercising
18. Being fearful, insecure	Seeking love, not food
19. Snacking that is not planned	Planning between-meal snacks
20. Raiding refrigerator at night	"Reaching for your mate instead of your plate"
21. Sneaking cake or other goodies	Imagining these are covered with ants
22. Oversocializing	Planning for eating out or company; planning activities, games, or hobbies instead of eating during socializing

The fourth and final step is the decision to do something about your weight problem. Your aching back, as well as your overall health, will thank you!

1200-Calorie Meal Selections

As we have discussed, the average person burns approximately 2200 calories in a day and calories over this amount are turned into fat and extra weight. If your back pain has limited your physical activities, you may burn fewer than 2200 calories. The following 1200-calorie menus are designed to help you gradually lose extra pounds and keep them off. The menus consist of a 300-calorie breakfast, 400-calorie lunch, and 500-calorie dinner.

Breakfast

		Calories
Menu 1— 2 slices of bacon (press out grease)	86	
1 egg cooked to your preference	80	
1 slice toast	65	
1 teaspoon of low-calorie jelly	32	
½ orange	35	
	298	calories
Menu 2— 1 cup dry cereal or ½ cup oatmeal	100	
1 teaspoon sugar	15	
½ cup of skim milk	44	
1 cup of tomato juice	45	
1 banana	102	
	306	calories

Lunch

Menu 1— Hamburger (lean ground beef)	355	
1 peach	40	
	395	calories
Menu 2— Roast beef sandwich with lettuce,		
tomato, and mayonnaise	348	
½ orange	35	
	383	calories

Dinner

Menu 1— Steak (broiled)	240	
1 small baked potato	93	
1 teaspoon of sour cream	26	
1 cup of green beans (steamed)	30	
1 slice of bread	65	
½ cup fresh strawberries	35	
	489	calories
Menu 2— Fried chicken (½ breast)	232	
Green peas	56	
1 cup of green beans (steamed)	30	
1 cup of ice cream	193	
	511	calories

It is a good idea to consult your physician before beginning a diet to ask his or her opinion of other sound dieting principles and ideas for a wider variety of food selections. *Stay away from fad diets that promise rapid weight loss!* While on some fad diets you may lose weight rapidly but what they don't tell you is that the initial weight loss is probably 80 percent water and there is very little water in fat. Water loss comes primarily from blood and muscles, which explains part of why you are likely to feel so weak after several days on a fad diet. Furthermore, as soon as you return to your normal eating pattern, you will gain the lost fluids back and you will still have the same amount of fat. Keep in mind that to lose weight and keep it off, you must reduce the number of calories you eat or increase your exercise and activity level or *both*!

Diet Drugs

Almost all of us who have sought to lose weight have considered using diet pills. While some people realize the potential danger of this approach, an alarming number do not. Dieters spend over $170 million per year for diet drugs. A panel of experts for the Food and Drug Administration (FDA) periodically reviews all nonprescription drugs sold for weight control. The panel recently found that most ingredients now being sold over the counter for this purpose have *not* been shown to be safe and effective.

Diet drugs, prescription or nonprescription, are classified as (1) anorexiants, (2) bulk-forming agents, and (3) topical or local anesthetics. Before you invest your money and trust your health to these drugs, you should know the answers to these three questions: How do they work? Are they effective? Are they safe?

Anorexiants decrease food intake by interfering with brain hormones. A section of the brain called the hypothalamus tells you when you are hungry and when you are full and anorexiants act on this region of the brain. Unfortunately tolerance soon develops to this class of drugs and they become ineffective at recommended drug dosages. Do not use these drugs without first consulting your doctor, particularly if you suffer from diabetes, heart disease, high blood pressure, or thyroid disease. An aching back is enough of a problem without adding to your misery.

Bulk-forming agents are used in some nonprescription products. The idea is that they produce a feeling of fullness, thus reducing the desire to eat. Recent studies indicate that the feeling of fullness passes in less than 30 minutes and that these drugs may also have a very harsh laxative effect.

Local anesthetics, such as benzocaine, are also frequently found in weight-control preparations. Proponents claim that this drug class suppresses appetite by reducing our sensitivity to taste. There is, however, no conclusive evidence to prove that local anesthetics are effective in weight control and individuals who take these drugs over periods of time expose themselves to drug-induced allergic reactions, such as skin rash and shortness of breath.

Beware of diet drugs! The safest and most effective way to reduce weight and take a heavy load off of your aching back is to decrease caloric intake and increase physical exercise.

NUTRITION

In addition to how much we eat, what we eat has been repeatedly documented as important for our overall health. Studies also suggest that various foods and nutrients can have an effect on the amount of pain and discomfort we experience—which is particularly interesting news for the back pain victim!

What Everyone Should Know About Nutrition

To meet our body needs, an adequate diet must provide all known nutrients and, no doubt, a few more still to be discovered. The 50 or so known nutrients include proteins, fats, carbohydrates, vitamins, minerals, and water. Although they are widely distributed in our foods, no single food contains all of the nutrients we need.

Nutritionists have divided the nutrients we need for good health into four basic food groups. The average adult can very simply meet the recommended dietary allowance by consuming daily two servings from the milk group, five ounces from the meat group, four servings from the bread group, and four from the vegetable–fruit group.

The *meat group* contains meats, poultry, fish, eggs, and legumes such as dried beans, peas, and nuts. All are good sources of protein, and also supply needed B-complex vitamins.

Unfortunately meat adds calories, fat, and cholesterol to the diet in rather large quantities and much of the fat in meat is of the saturated type. Since saturated fat and cholesterol are linked with development of coronary heart disease, portion sizes of meat to be consumed should be limited.

The *bread and cereal group* is often misunderstood and inaccurately reported as being fattening, overprocessed, and full of additives. This is simply not true! Bread and cereal are valuable sources of important nutrients, some of which are difficult to obtain without including this group. Of course, moderation with any food group is important.

Milk and milk products provide more calcium than any other food and also supply the body with valuable protein and vitamins. Weight-conscious consumers often seem to omit milk products from their daily diets because of calorie counting. The new low-fat milks, with fewer calories and less cholesterol, or fat-free skim milk is a good solution.

The *fruit and vegetable group* is probably the most neglected, and yet most important, of the food groups. Research has indicated that our diets are most often deficient in vitamin C, 90 percent of which is provided by the fruit and vegetable group. Vitamin A is often found to be in short supply in the diets of our older citizens and fruits and vegetables provide 60 percent of vitamin A.

Few can deny that nutrition is related in some manner to every aspect of human health, growth, and development. An aching back requires that every other part of our body be as strong and healthy as possible if we are to win the battle against pain. Yet, Americans seem to ignore nutritional health as much as the well-being of our backs.

If our nutritional ignorance has resulted from lack of food education, then we have the responsibility to ensure that the present school-age population does not grow up with the same misinformation, confusion, and ignorance. Among other things we can support the 1972 recommendation of the National Advisory Council on Child Nutrition, which favored "nutritional education as a curriculum component for all grades in elementary and secondary schools, and that nutrition courses be required for teacher certification."

Nutritional Pain Control?

Over the past several years, a small flurry of interest has been generated by several scientists researching the effects of controlling chronic pain through nutrition. Receiving the most attention has been a common amino acid called *phenylalanine*. Since proteins in the body are made from amino acids, these acids serve a valuable bodily function. Phenylalanine is available in many of the foods we eat, as well as in over-the-counter tablets. It comes in three forms. L- (or laevo) phenylalanine is the form most commonly found in high-protein foods and is the type the body uses to make its own protein. D- (or dextro) phenylalanine is very similar to the "l" form but is found most abundantly in bacteria and plant tissue. The human body slowly converts d-phenylalanine to l-phenylalanine before it is utilized in known bodily functions. The third kind is an equal mixture of the d and l forms and is referred to, naturally enough, as dl-phenylalanine or DLPA. DLPA is considered by some authorities to be a major breakthrough in the "natural" control of chronic pain.

In 1978 Dr. Seymour Ehrenpresis and others from the department of pharmacology and anesthesiology at the University of Chicago Medical School published the results of a chemical study of d-phenylalanine (DPA) in the treatment of various chronic pain conditions. The first patient had suffered from whiplash pain for two years and had previously been treated with various medications without relief. After taking DPA for two days, the patient reported complete pain relief that lasted for one month after he had stopped taking the amino acid and no adverse side effects were reported. Other patients who were successfully treated with DPA had low back pain problems and arthritis. A subsequent study by these researchers found that 75 percent of chronic pain patients responded favorably to DPA administration. Some experienced marked relief within the first week; others required up to four weeks before significant relief was achieved.

Since the initial discovery, pain research has concentrated on using the "dl" form of phenylalanine since it has a greater nutritive value for the body.

How does DLPA work? Investigators suggest that it reduces chronic pain by intensifying and prolonging the body's own natural pain-killing response. You will recall from Chapter 3 our discussion of the body's own morphinelike hormones naturally produced in response to pain signals received in the brain. Research has indicated that many chronic pain patients have significantly lower levels of endorphin activity in their blood and cerebrospinal fluid as compared with individuals who do not suffer pain. DLPA is thought by some to restore endorphin hormone levels to a normal range, which theoretically produces a reduction in pain and discomfort.

Does DLPA really reduce the intensity of chronic pain? My frankest answer is—I don't know! Some researchers and scientists strongly believe in the value of DLPA whereas other health care professionals either remain unconvinced or even laugh at the absurdity of the idea. We do know that studies on the pain-reducing potential of DLPA are in their infancy and no well-controlled, large-scale studies have been conducted to date. Until such convincing research is forthcoming, the use of supplemental DLPA must be considered *experimental.*

But if your aching back is saying that you cannot wait, discuss DLPA with your physician. Tablets are generally available at health food stores and drugstores.

SLEEP

Have you ever spent a night tossing and turning and unable to sleep? Remember the irritating darkness and how the minutes crawled? Remember the frustration that built as you fought without success to get comfortable and sleep? Remember the groggy, washed-out feeling the following morning?

Practically everyone has experienced an occasional sleepless night. But some people, chronic back pain sufferers, find that sleepless nights are the rule rather than the exception. Of the back pain patients treated at our centers, 94 percent either report problems with falling asleep, with staying asleep, or both. And while an occasional restless night is little to be concerned about, chronic sleep problems can have devastating effects. Sleep deprivation results in mounting irritability, frustration, fatigue, depression, anxiety, and a host of other emotional and physical effects. While persons in pain, as well as those who work with patients in pain, need no documentation of this fact, sleep deprivation studies over the past years have repeatedly evidenced the profound nervous system drain caused by chronic sleep problems. And if you recall the feedback loop of pain described throughout this text, it is easy to see how increased irritability, frustration, fatigue, depression, and anxiety create a state of heightened physiological arousal in the body that further increases the pain. As pain increases, sleep problems also intensify in a cyclic fashion. Sleep problems may not cause back discomfort but can certainly make a distressing discomfort much more agonizing.

What is the answer for getting a good night's sleep? Sleeping pills? How about a glass of warm milk or maybe alcohol? How about a late-night snack?

The Rhythm of Sleep

Sleep occurs in five stages. In stage I an individual is still somewhat aware of the surroundings but is very relaxed and dreamy. In this stage a person may jerk involuntarily and wake up in the process. Stage I sleep only lasts a few minutes.

Stages II and III mean progressively deeper levels of sleep, but though unaware of the surroundings, the person wakes easily. Approximately 40 minutes after the onset of stage I, stage IV begins. This is a state of profound sleep from which arousal is difficult. There is little body movement during this stage and pulse, respiration, and blood pressure decrease. This is what most people think of as sleep, and they tend to assess the adequacy of their sleep on the basis of how long they believe they were in this deep stage of oblivion.

Stage IV restores, relaxes, and rests the body physically. After strenuous physical activity, the need for stage IV sleep is greater. Following a day of heavy physical exertion, a person is likely to awaken with the feeling of having slept long and soundly. Stage IV is only one type of sleep, however, and does not meet all sleep needs.

By the end of about 90 minutes, one gradually returns through the lighter stages of sleep to stage I. Instead of reentering stage I or waking at this time, one enters the stage of REM (rapid eye movement) sleep, and then proceeds back through stages II, III, and IV again.

REM sleep has many unique features, such as frequent bursts of rapid eye movement, which can be observed through closed eyelids, muscular twitching, dreams, and profound muscular relaxation. In addition to the rapid eye movement, REM sleep may be recognized by the complete relaxation of the lower jaw. The pulse becomes irregular and blood pressure is variable. Males of all ages have penile erections during REM sleep and stomach secretion is increased in both sexes.

Some people are concerned when they dream because they think it means that their sleep was not as sound as it should be. However, studies of sleep behavior reveal that everyone dreams during REM sleep, although the dreams may not be remembered. What about the content of those rich REM stage dreams? That, of course, is a matter for much speculation.

Some scientists have postulated that dreams are nothing more than random flashes of the brain the reasoning portion of the mind attempts to interpret logically. In essence the brain fires and we draw on stored memories to make sense of the "thoughts."

One interesting note: As the night wears on, we apparently draw on images stored deeper and deeper. Childhood memories predominate in the dreams during predawn REM sleep.

Other researchers have suggested that dreams are heavily influenced by both the previous day's activity and external forces at work while you dream. A steady diet of spy films before you fall asleep may inspire a "spy" dream. In one experiment sleepers wore "rose-colored glasses" during all their waking hours. Their subsequent dreams were primarily in red, although normal dreams generally show a preponderance of the color green, followed by blue, yellow, and red.

What goes on while we sleep is also important. If you are sprayed with water while you sleep (another experiment that has been done in the sleep lab), you will have a dream in which liquids play a part. Similarly, if your covers are off, you may dream of cold. Factory whistles can become trains, snoring can transform into a motorcycle, or the radio turn into a live band or just a radio.

Such images as flying, spinning, or floating, which in the past have given rise to involved interpretation, may in fact be nothing more than a reflection of the heavy muscle suppression that accompanies REM sleep. By the same token, frequent dreams about being in your pajamas or nude may not be sexual at all, but more a reflection of the state of your nighttime dress.

Everyone goes through an average of four or five cycles of sleep each night, each lasting from 90 to 100 minutes. Stage IV decreases and REM sleep increases progressively with each cycle, so that most stage IV sleep occurs early in the night and most REM sleep during the last few hours before rising. The REM stage of the first cycle is only a few minutes, but 25 percent of the total sleep time is REM sleep. People generally are aware that they sleep more lightly and dream more during the hours just before waking.

A Good Night Equals a Good Day

Remember how your mother struggled to get you to bed when you were a child with the promise (among assorted threats) that a good night equals a good day? Well, Mom was right again! Sleep studies have consistently reported that frustration, irritation, anxiety, depression, and increased back pain result from inadequate sleep. But how do you get a good night's sleep when your back hurts and every movement sends shooting pain throughout your body? I can suggest some "do's" that may work for you, but first let us eliminate some "don'ts."

First, do not rely on pills for sound and restful sleep. Sleeping pills consistently derange the body's natural sleep process and may suppress one or more of the essential stages of sleep (stage IV or REM). When this happens you may "technically" sleep, but the sleep will not be restful or refreshing and you will feel groggy and fatigued the following day. Furthermore, there is growing scientific evidence suggesting that most sleeping pills alter the composition of one or more of our natural body chemicals that control (to some degree) our sensitivity to pain. In other words, taking sleeping pills may cause us to experience back pain more acutely and severely than we otherwise would. In addition, using such pills over a period of time is thought to force the body into a dependence on chemically induced sleep. We lose our natural ability to rest. Take away the sleeping aid and we find that our bodies have "forgotten" how to go to sleep "naturally." This may result in nightmares and further restlessness and fatigue.

Second, some foods contain stimulants that alter the natural cycle and interfere with the orderly progression from one sleep stage to the next. Coffee and tea are well-known stimulants; lesser known may be the cola drinks or that often praised cup of hot chocolate before bedtime. Certain spicy foods (in fact, any large meal too close to bedtime) can alter sleep patterns. So, too, can stomach-rattling hunger.

Third, you can also upset the sleep cycle through excessive thinking. Worry can cause the body to release chemicals every bit as bothersome as caffeine. Even mild anxiety and nervousness can cause the mind to resist the relaxation needed to fall into a deep sleep. The old advice "Never go to bed angry!" has been borne out by sleep research.

Finally, many people believe that an alcoholic drink before retiring assists in sleeping. The truth is that while alcohol may speed the onset of sleep, it greatly interferes with REM sleep. The hangover that so often follows alcohol consumption may be partially due to REM deprivation.

Now that we know what to avoid, how about some hints for improved sleep, especially sleeping with a painful back?

The *progressive relaxation exercise* outlined in Chapter 11 is critically important. Go back and review the mechanics of this most valuable relaxing, pain-controlling, and sleep-inducing technique and remember the importance of practicing this skill several times each day. Remember, also, that progressive relaxation is a skill that not only must be learned but also must be practiced in order to become more proficient.

The next chapter in this book explains and illustrates the importance of proper body posture and body mechanics in controlling back pain. Pay particular attention to the section on sleeping. Proper posture while sleeping can reduce much of the pressure and strain on the back and thereby reduce pain. If you have difficulty going to sleep or wake during the night due to back pain, this discussion may help.

Although no definitive evidence exists to support the old remedy of drinking a glass of warm milk at bedtime to promote sleep, there is some justification for its use. Most protein foods, including milk and some vegetables, contain the amino acid *L-tryptophan*. L-tryptophan is closely related to one of the body's natural chemicals believed to induce and maintain sleep. In doses as low as one gram, it has been found to speed the onset and prolong the period of sleep without altering the REM sleep or sleep rhythms in any way. Even in much larger doses, no serious side effects have been noted to date.

Eight glasses of milk would be needed to provide one gram of L-tryptophan, but it is possible that the small amount contained in a single glass might be sufficient to make a difference in sleep. It is also possible that the amount contained in a glass of milk added to the person's L-tryptophan intake at dinner will enhance sleep. It has been speculated that the L-tryptophan content of certain foods partially explains why we are sometimes sleepy after eating a heavy meal.

Finally, keep in mind that there is no such thing as "can't sleep." You may have trouble falling asleep, staying asleep, or sleeping during selected times, but when your body reaches a certain state of sleep deprivation, you will go to sleep, back pain or no back pain. You may reach this state in the middle of a working day, in the course of an important conversation, or in what we generally consider as sleeping hours, but you *will* go to sleep sooner or later. Most back pain victims who complain that they "can't sleep" are really saying that they do not go to sleep when they wish or stay asleep as long as they would choose. This being the case, your job is to work to *improve* your sleep by following the suggestions outlined above. It may take time and effort but the results in improved sleep are worth the trouble.

You can win the battle against back pain and its associated miseries!

14

THE BACK SCHOOL: BODY POSTURE
FOR BACK PAIN RELIEF

I happened to watch a rerun of the old *Star Trek* television series several months ago on cable television. In this particular episode, Mr. Scott had been attacked by a band of hostile inhabitants of an unknown star. Poor Scotty had quite a time and received multiple and serious injuries, particularly to the arms and chest. But thanks to the science fiction of space-age medicine, Dr. McCoy was successful in diagnosing Scotty's injuries with a hand-held scanner and subsequently closing the open wounds with a laser beam device carried on the belt. You will be relieved to know that Mr. Scott was as good as new before Captain Kirk and Mr. Spock had even decided on appropriate punishment for this unprovoked transgression.

As I watched the *Enterprise* "boldly go where no man had gone before," I couldn't help but wonder how this scenario might have differed had Mr. Scott injured his back in the tussle. I can imagine Dr. McCoy's look of resignation when he admitted to Scotty that even space-age medicine had no total and rapid cure for the aching back. I can even imagine Dr. McCoy instructing Mr. Scott that the responsibility for managing the intensity of his back pain and living a productive life was a personal one that the valued technician himself must assume. Even the unbridled artistic license of space fiction must occasionally be tempered with the harsh reality that there exists no magic or technological miracle cure for the chronically painful back.

Making the decision to assume primary responsibility for the care of your aching back is mandatory for successful pain management. This decision is the foundation of the Tollison Program. Relief may not come as quickly as a magic blast from Dr. McCoy's space-age laser, but it will be lasting and you will feel and look better. But as pointed out in the preceding chapters, the decision to participate fully in the program is yours to make.

The present chapter is based on and credited to the love and guidance of mothers around the world. Remember your mother's encouragement to "take care of your body and it will take care of you"? Well, guess what? Your mother was right, again!

Think about your relationship with your back. How have you treated your back over the years? Have you cared for and protected your back? Have you treated it with the respect and consideration worthy of such a hard-working friend? If you treated your next-door neighbor in the same manner that you have treated your back over the years, would your neighbor now be a helpful and assisting friend or an irritating and frustrating enemy?

Many victims of chronic back pain have a lengthy history of back abuse. Regardless of whether the actual pain started gradually or with some identified accident or trauma, a history of back abuse remains generally true. Perhaps this abuse has taken the form of inconsideration and neglect. Most of us give our teeth protection by brushing and regular dental examinations. Most of us also give our hearts protective consideration by avoiding fatty foods and smoking, while engaging in some type of regular exercise. So why do we ignore the back until the cumulative effects of neglect and abuse result in an intensity of discomfort sufficient to capture our attention? Regrettably, we spend hours each day standing, sitting, sleeping, lifting, bending, reaching, and driving but seldom stop to consider what effect these repetitive motions have on our backs.

Seldom do our bodies allow us the privilege of lengthy negative treatment without ultimately paying the price. In fact, even our tolerant and strong friend the back will only accept so much before complaining. And if you suffer the aching, burning misery of back pain, I need not remind you of how intensely the back can protest!

If you have been remiss in the proper care of your back and now suffer spinal revenge, there is no time like the present to modify your attitude and habits. The first step is to consider the back. This chapter will show you proper posture and body mechanics to use at work, home, and play. It will also show you other ways to be considerate of your back 24 hours a day. The second step is to think ahead. One of the most important habits you can develop is to use your *mind* before you use your *body*. Read this chapter carefully and practice implementing the body mechanics demonstrated. In many ways this chapter is like an "owner's manual" that explains the correct use of the back. The techniques and body mechanics illustrated are an important part of the Tollison Program for back pain relief and are regularly taught in our PAIN THERAPY CENTERS℠ Back School and Strengthening Program. They can work for you, too!

STANDING

Slouchers are easy targets for back trouble. When the shoulders are slumped, the pelvis tilts forward, the ribs point downward, the chin is out, and the lower spine is swayback. This posture not only crowds and pushes the internal organs together, but it also may strain muscles and ligaments in the spine.

Just as slouching or slumping is asking for back trouble, so too is the exaggerated military posture many of us were told was the correct way to stand. Such a posture forces the shoulders too far back, and the muscles are held too tightly. The worst part, however, is the curve that this rigid posture creates in the small of the back.

The best way to stand is relaxed, with your head straight, chin slightly tucked, stomach in, and the buttocks tucked under. While the spine is never perfectly straight, this relaxed posture, combined with a slight backward tilt, straightens the spine to its most natural curve and also provides relief from ligament and muscle strain.

When you must stand for long intervals, put one foot on a stool. Every few minutes put the other foot up; alternate. Prolonged standing fatigues the hip muscles and slowly pulls the pelvis forward. This creates an unnatural curve in the lower spine and strains the lower back mucles. Placing a foot on a stool counteracts this stress by returning the spine to its natural shape.

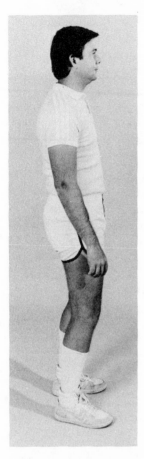

Photograph 14-1—Proper body mechanics when standing can decrease ligament and muscle strain and provide a welcomed reduction in back pain.

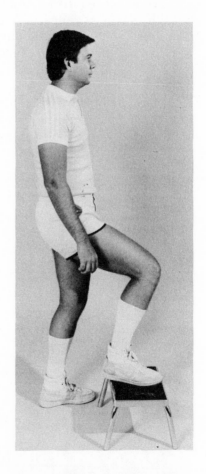

Photograph 14-2—Placing one foot on a stool when standing pulls the pelvis and lower back into a neutral position.

SITTING

Sitting is more stressful to your back than standing because the spine is no longer balanced on the pelvis. When one is seated, the pelvis tends to tilt backwards, flattening the normal curve of the lower spine. After a period of time, ligaments and muscles in the back begin to protest. Avoid stuffy chairs that sink in with your weight to mold your body shape. It is also best to avoid chairs that force you to sit in awkward positions.

If your job requires a great deal of sitting, choose a chair that hugs the small of your back. Adjust the height of the chair so that your knees are level with or slightly higher than your hips, and keep both feet flat on the floor. Crossing your legs tilts the pelvis forward much the same way that prolonged standing does and is murder on the back.

Never sit for more than an hour without walking around and stretching. Balancing the books of a multimillion-dollar company or the family checkbook requires intense concentration and creates

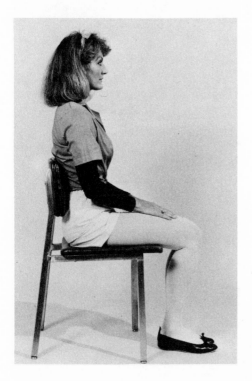

Photograph 14-3
—Improper sitting posture can create additional low back stress and pain.

generalized muscle tension. A quick walk every hour to the office water fountain or the family kitchen will help relax your muscles and your mind.

Driving an automobile can also be hazardous to your back if you do not sit properly. Adjust the seat so that your feet can reach the pedals without stretching your legs. Sports cars are built low to the ground and require that your legs be straight, thus straining the muscles in the lower back. If you drive a lot, buy a firm supportive backrest. It is also a good idea to pull off the road every hour or so to get out of the car and stretch. Your back will thank you!

SLEEPING

The key to proper sleeping habits is the knees. Bending the knees unlocks the spine into a neutral position and relieves ligament and muscle stress. Since most of us spend as much as one-third of our lives sleeping, proper sleeping posture is very important in the care of the back.

Start with a firm mattress. As in sitting, the spine should be supported in a neutral position. This requires a firm mattress to prevent sagging. It is not necessary to buy a special orthopedic mattress unless your doctor recommends it. Almost any mattress can be made firm enough by putting a plywood board under it.

There are two proper positions for sleeping. The first is on your back. If you are comfortable sleeping on your back, place a pillow or cushion under your knees to bend the knees. This will neutralize the swayback that is created when you lie flat with your legs straight.

If you are most comfortable on your side, this position is fine, too. Use a pillow under your head so that your neck is properly aligned with your spine. Next bent the knees to neutralize spinal stress and place a pillow between the knees to keep from twisting the lower back.

Now some "don'ts" about proper sleeping posture. First, don't sleep on your stomach. This position causes swayback and increased muscle and ligament stress. Second, don't sleep on a waterbed. Waterbeds do not provide proper firmness and support for the spine. Finally, don't prop yourself up to read in bed. This causes an unnatural curve in the spine and spells disaster for the back.

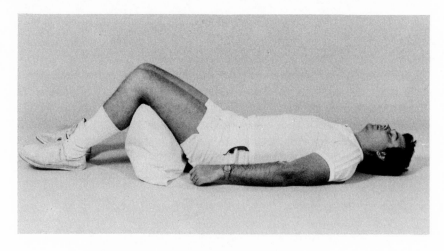

Photograph 14-4—Bending the knees releases your back into a more neutral position.

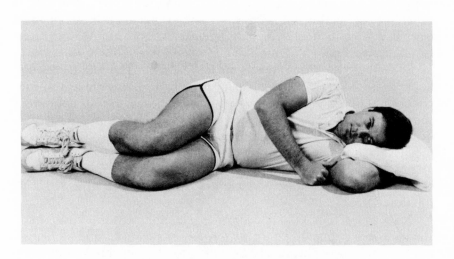

Photograph 14-5—Given the length of time that is spent sleeping, proper body mechanics is a must for proper spinal care.

LIFTING

Probably more back injuries result from improper lifting than from any other activity. Since most backaches result from minor injuries, careful lifting will eliminate many problems.

When lifting, let the legs do the work. Weightlifters know the proper posture for lifting is bending the knees and keeping the back straight. Position your body with one foot ahead of the other for balance and pull the object close to your body before lifting it. If you bend from the waist with your legs straight, you may some day find it impossible to get back up again! Grasp the object firmly and lift with the legs, keeping the object close to the body and lifting it no higher than your waist. Never turn from the waist. Instead, turn from the feet or point the forward foot in the direction of the turn in order to reduce twisting of the body. Heavy objects should be set down the same way.

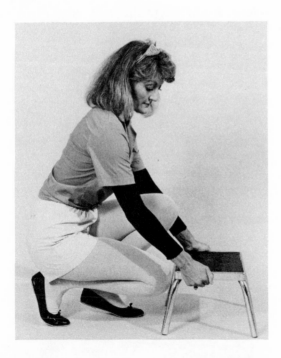

Photograph 14-6—When bending, let the legs do the work. Muscles in the legs are much less prone to injury than the lower back.

Think about your back when lifting luggage, tying shoes, or raking leaves. Never reach into the back seat or trunk of a car to lift a heavy suitcase. When tying your shoes, squat rather than bend at the waist. Finally, rake leaves from left to right or right to left; never stretch forward to pull the leaves toward your feet.

BENDING

Bending at the waist should be avoided whenever possible since bending throws the distribution of body weight off balance. Body weight is balanced on the pelvis, which acts as a fulcrum for the upper and lower body. Bending tilts this balance and places a strain on the disks, muscles, and ligaments that support the spine.

What do you do if you drop the car keys on the floor? *Squat* rather than bend, keeping the back in a vertical position. Squatting uses the leg muscles rather than the back muscles. Since muscles

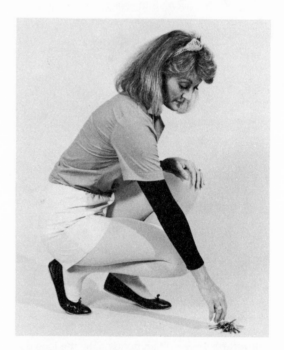

Photograph 14-7—A good habit to develop is to squat rather than bend!

in the lower back may be no larger than your finger and those in the legs may be as large as your wrist, squatting can prevent a painful back injury.

When you buy a new vacuum cleaner, take it for a practice spin and check to see if you can use it without stooping. If you are already saddled with the wrong kind, bend your knees slightly while vacuuming rather than stooping over. If you decide to do some minor mechanical repairs on your car, lie across the fender rather than bend over it, especially if you are not accustomed to regularly bending over an automobile engine. While making beds, do a few knee bends to tuck in the corners and walk around the bed. Don't reach for the opposite corner of a queen-sized bed. Finally, adjust the lawn mower handles to your height, so you need not bend over to grasp them.

You may be very pleasantly surprised at the noticeable reduction in back pain that results from practicing proper body mechanics. I once saw a new patient referred to me after more than three decades of low back and leg pain. Mr. X had been hospitalized eight times for diagnosis and treatment of his pain. He estimated that the combination of hospitalization and home bed rest had resulted in his missing more than two years from work in his 31-year history of back pain.

During my routine intake interview, I learned that Mr. X was an attorney who spend most of each day sitting at his desk. I questioned him about his chair and learned that it did not allow the proper posture of knees higher than the hips. In fact, the chair was an antique piece previously owned by the patient's father and provided very poor support of the lower back.

I contemplated hospitalizing Mr. X for an intensive back rehabilitation program (see Chapter 15) but elected instead to try a two-week experiment. After a full explanation of the science of body mechanics with particular emphasis on sitting posture, I sent Mr. X home with the suggestion that he purchase and use a desk chair that positioned his knees slightly higher than the level of his hips. After a two-week trial, he was to return to my office for evaluation.

Nine days later I received a telephone call from an excited Mr. X who reported the complete elimination of the back and leg pain that had plagued him for so many years. When I last saw him a year later, his pain was still a problem of the past and he was a strong proponent of body mechanics and proper posture.

While you may not experience the dramatic elimination of back pain that Mr. X did, it is a near certainty that the daily and consistent practice of proper body mechanics will make a positive difference in your pain intensity. And if you incorporate body mechanics with the other components of the Tollison Program described in this book, the chances are excellent that you are on your way to improved back pain management.

What if you faithfully follow the program outlined and still are unable to function due to severe back discomfort? Unfortunately a small percentage of those reading this book may find this to be the case. If so, do not despair. The chances are excellent that you simply need the added intensiveness, structure, and comprehensiveness available in a hospital-based interdisciplinary pain clinic. But let the buyer beware! Pain clinics vary greatly in terms of scope, effectiveness, and competency. In Chapter 15 we will examine the characteristics that you should look for in choosing a good pain clinic, and explain what you can expect from interdisciplinary and intensive pain control treatment.

15

PAIN CLINICS: WHAT THEY CAN DO FOR YOU

What is a pain clinic? It is just about any place that wants to call itself one. There has been a pain clinic explosion in the United States since 1976, when a national survey counted 17 of them. No one is sure how many pain treatment programs exist today, but educated guesses range from 500 to more than 1000. The clinics range from nonlicensed or weakly licensed "quacks" to interdisciplinary programs involving clinical psychologists, neurosurgeons, orthopedic surgeons, anesthesiologists, physical therapists, occupational therapists, recreational therapists, biofeedback technicians, vocational counselors, rehabilitation nurses, and others.

While practically anything or anyone can be called a pain clinic, interdisciplinary pain treatment programs are undoubtedly the "state of the art." The reason is simple: No *simple* treatment technique is as likely to aid in the control of your back pain as is a combination of therapies. Chronic back pain is a multifaceted problem; consequently, effective treatment is best accomplished with a multifaceted or interdisciplinary approach.

The best pain clinics are interdisciplinary both in treatment and in staff. This simply means that a number of different doctors and therapists, representing a variety of specialties and skilled in a range of treatments, work together with you toward successful back pain control. One example of interdisciplinary treatment is this book. Think of the various treatments that we have discussed—medications, manipulations, relaxation training, ice therapy, and physical exercise, just to name a few. Combine all of these therapies and you have an interdisciplinary pain management program. Approximately 35–40 programs in the United States fit this description.

If you suffer chronic back pain, you know that your condition is far more complex than the discomfort alone. In addition to the pain, many suffer disrupted marital and family relationships, vocational disability, loss of or decreased financial income, drug dependence or addiction, depression, anxiety, reduced sense of self-worth and self-esteem, deconditioned physical states, and other assorted physical, social, and psychological problems. These are symptoms of the disease of chronic back pain and are common to most sufferers. Since professional attention to only one or two of these problems will leave the other symptoms festering and continuing to result in back misery, a more intensive and comprehensive effort may be needed to reverse the negative and deteriorating spiral of chronic back pain. In this age of "superspecialists," an interdisciplinary team approach assures that *all* aspects of the pain will receive professional attention. Thus an interdisciplinary and intensive approach may offer you the best chance for back pain relief.

Do you need a comprehensive interdisciplinary pain clinic for back pain control? Perhaps. The techniques described in this book are presented because they have proved effective in reducing back pain. But if your pain persists after faithfully following the program outlined, it is likely that an interdisciplinary pain treatment center will provide the greater intensity of treatment necessary to reverse the problem. The treatments may be similar to the techniques described here, but more comprehensive and intense. In addition, these treatment centers will have specially trained doctors to administer selective therapies that require professional involvement.

Generally, an interdisciplinary pain treatment center should be considered in the following circumstances:

1. You have suffered back pain for longer than six months.
2. You take medication for pain control.
3. You are vocationally disabled or miss more than one week of work each year because of back pain.
4. You are unable to enjoy hobbies and recreational activities because of pain.
5. You have had back surgery without pain relief or have been told that back surgery may be necessary in the future.
6. You suffer sleep distress as a result of your pain.
7. You have faithfully tried the treatment techniques described in this book and have experienced at least some relief for your back discomfort.

What can you expect from treatment at a pain clinic? It is impossible to describe this specifically since treatment centers vary greatly with regard to technique, procedure, staffing, and philosophy. Pain treatment centers may be inpatient or outpatient facilities, may function with no doctors or with a staff of specialists, may administer one type of treatment or employ an interdisciplinary team approach to treatment, may accept every patient who wanders through the door or intensively evaluate each patient referred to ensure that specialized treatment is appropriate, and so on.

A solution to describing such a wide variety of programs is to describe one model program. As founder and director of the interdisciplinary PAIN THERAPY CENTERS℠ clinical programs located in numerous hospitals, the outline of pain clinic treatment that is presented in this chapter is limited to a description of our approach to the rehabilitation of chronic back pain sufferers.

THE PAIN THERAPY CENTERS

PAIN THERAPY CENTERS℠ began in 1980 in Greenville, S.C. At that time the Greenville Hospital System had a desire to provide a quality treatment program for the victims of intractable pain served by the hospital, and a young specialist in clinical psychology and behavioral medicine was recruited who had a number of unique ideas and theories with regard to chronic pain management. The association has been good, additional programs have opened in various cities to serve the needs of individuals suffering chronic pain, and thousands of pain sufferers have been treated in these programs.

What accounts for the success of this clinical treatment? There are numerous reasons, many of which can be found in the treatment program described throughout this book. But perhaps most important is the clinical philosophy that chronic pain, including intractable back pain, seldom results from a single, isolated cause. The uniqueness of our centers' clinical services and the Tollison Program lies in the fact that chronic back pain is a *biphasic* or *psychophysiologic* component. Intractable back pain may start with a slip, twist, accident, fall, or disease. Muscles may be torn or strained, a disk may herniate or a vertebra may fracture, or more than 100 other *physical* causes may initially start the cycle of painful misery.

But the physical cause of pain does not fully explain the total discomfort and misery involved. If chronic back pain is solely a physical problem, then why do physical treatments and remedies alone so seldom result in relief? Why do physical treatment modalities such as muscle relaxants and anti-inflammatory drugs, ultrasound, bed rest, back braces, traction, and other physical treatments so rarely bring relief to victims who have suffered months and years of back misery? Why does back surgery fail to help three of every four back pain victims who elect to undergo it? If chronic back pain is only a physical problem, then why do we see the number of chronic back pain victims increase every year, reaching epidemic proportions, despite continued advances and greater sophistication in physical diagnosis and treatment?

The answer lies in the fact that chronic back pain is more than just a physical problem. It is a biphasic problem, composed of both physical and psychological components. Medications, ultrasound, traction, surgery, and other physical treatments may eliminate or reduce the physical component of pain, but they do not address the *psychological* or emotional component of back pain. As a result the back continues to hurt and the victim remains in misery.

What is needed is recognition and acceptance that chronic back pain is a psychophysiologic problem, and only a comprehensive, interdisciplinary rehabilitation program is designed to address *all* aspects of the pain problem. PAIN THERAPY CENTERS℠ is founded on this philosophy, and results have been favorable:

1. Reduced subjective pain intensity of 31 percent.
2. Increase in physical activity of 343 percent.
3. Reduction in medication usage of 88 percent.
4. Reduction in health care utilization of 76 percent.
5. Return to productive employment of 64 percent.

What can you expect if you are referred by your doctor to one of our programs? Our treatment is designed for selected patients who have suffered persisting pain for longer than six months without satisfactory response to traditional medical treatment. The "average" pain patient may be described as suffering from low back and/or neck pain as the result of an injury (although other types of pain are treated); unemployed or physically and/or psychologically disabled, having undergone as many as seven major operations for pain relief; habituated to or dependent on narcotic medication; experiencing serious and significant depression; demonstrating a loss of interest in physical, vocational, and social activities; and suffering a breakdown in family and interpersonal relationships.

Our programs are designed to counteract the disabling effects of chronic pain. Treatment is interdisciplinary and comprehensive as each therapy interrelates during the average 25-day inpatient hospitalization. The primary treatment team includes a medical psychologist/behavioral medicine specialist, behavior therapists, physical therapists, physicians, social workers, vocational rehabilitation counselors, recreational therapists, and rehabilitation nurses. Consultants representing neurosurgery, orthopedic surgery, and other specialty areas offer specialized services as needed.

Treatment in our programs is *not* the passive servicing of sick persons found in acute or general hospitals, but is active, goal oriented, and directive (Table 15-1). Treatment rewards "wellness" and independence as the patient and staff actively work toward positive changes in the patient's physical and psychological lifestyle. The endless cycle of drugs, doctors, surgeries, suffering, and disability is broken as the patient is taught more effective means of pain control and, as a result, adopts a more active, productive, and independent style of living. Our treatment goals include:

1. Reduction of pain behavior in each patient.
2. Establishment and maintenance of effective well behavior.
3. Increase in frequency and extent of physical exercise and activity.
4. Reduction or elimination of medication intake.
5. Rearrangement of responses to both pain and well behavior by family and significant others (e.g., friends, employer, etc.).
6. Reduction of excessive health-care utilization.
7. Reduction of disability.
8. Return to work force (when appropriate).

While admission to some pain clinics is near automatic, patients referred to PAIN THERAPY CENTERS℠ programs are carefully evaluated and screened prior to acceptance. Preadmission evaluations involve comprehensive physical and psychological examinations, completion of questionnaires, and evaluations by physical, occupational, and recreational therapists, as well as social workers. Acceptance of treatment is contingent, in part, on the results of the preadmission evaluation and a belief by our staff members that you are truly motivated and determined to learn to manage your pain and resume a more productive lifestyle. Approximately one of every two patients evaluated is offered program admission. By concentrating on quality, rather than quantity, the intensive efforts required to reverse the downward spiral of chronic pain disability can be fully extended to every deserving patient.

TABLE 15-1

	MONDAY A	MONDAY B	TUESDAY A	TUESDAY B	WEDNESDAY A	WEDNESDAY B	THURSDAY A	THURSDAY B	FRIDAY A	FRIDAY B
8:30	Warmups PT		Warmups PT		Warmups PT		Warmups PT		Warmups PT	
9:00										
9:30	Group	Warmups PT	Voc Rehab	Warmups PT	Group	Warmups PT	Voc Rehab	Warmups PT	Group	Warmups PT
10:00										
10:30	Break Meds	Break Meds	Break Meds	Break Meds	Break Meds	Break Meds	Break Meds	Break Meds	Break Meds	Break Meds
11:00	Relaxation	Group	Relaxation	Voc Rehab	Relaxation	Group	Relaxation	Voc Rehab	Ice Massage	Group
11:30										
12:00	Lunch	Lunch	Lunch	Lunch	Lunch	Lunch	Lunch	Lunch	Lunch	Lunch
12:30										
1:00	Body Mechanics	Body Mechanics	Education	Relaxation	Body Mechanics	Body Mechanics	Education	Relaxation	Body Mechanics	Body Mechanics
1:30	PT	Relaxation	PT		PT	Relaxation	PT		PT	Ice Massage
2:00				Education				Education		
2:30	Break Meds	Break Meds	Break Meds	Break Meds	Break Meds	Break Meds	Break Meds	Break Meds	Break Meds	Break Meds
3:00	Pain School	Pain School	Pain School	Pain School	Pain School	Pain School	Pain School	Pain School	Pain School	Pain School
3:30										
4:00	End	PT	End	PT	End	PT	End	PT	End	PT
4:30										

TABLE 15-2
DAILY SCHEDULE

	SATURDAY	SUNDAY
7:00	Medications	Medications
8:00	Breakfast	Breakfast
8:30	Room Care	Room Care
9:00	Warm-Ups	Warm-Ups
9:30	Reconditioning Class	Reconditioning Class
10:30	Relaxation Training	Relaxation Training
11:00	Vocational Therapy	Vocational Therapy
12:00	Lunch	Lunch
1:00	Pass	Pass (earned)
10:00	Return	Return

PHYSICAL REHABILITATION

If you suffer chronic back pain, physical rehabilitation represents an important part of our treatment program, which is designed to reverse the negative spiral and deterioration of intractable pain and return you to a more enjoyable life-style. Approximately one-half of your rehabilitation program is carefully designed to aid in re-conditioning and strengthening you from the ground up! Many victims of chronic back pain lead a sedentary life, gain weight, develop tight muscles, and gradually become weakened and poorly conditioned. An important part of reducing your pain involves reversing this negative trend.

Realistic Expectations

In our programs, I generally see three types of back pain victims. Type 1 and type 2 are particularly difficult, while type 3 is primed for effective pain management treatment.

The first type wants, and practically demands, a total cure for the back misery. This type of patient does not want to discuss pain management, only pain elimination.

The second type of patient wants nothing and expects nothing. After suffering so much pain for so long, there are no expectations for improvement. This patient is depressed and has given up all hope, anticipating only continued pain and misery.

I would estimate the perhaps 80 percent of the patients I see in our treatment programs fall into one of these two general categories—chronic back pain sufferers with unrealistic and inappropriate expectations. Type 1 wants a total and permanent cure, and will accept nothing less. Type 2 is well-versed in self-fulfilling prophesy. This patient expects treatment failure and, as a result, generally gets it.

If you are a victim of chronic back pain, take a few moments to reconsider your expectations. Are you a type 1 patient, a type 2 patient, or a type 3 patient with realistic expectations? If you have suffered years of misery, have consulted numerous physicians, tried various treatments, including one or more failed back surgeries, and continue to suffer, your expectations for relief *must* be realistic. Treatment at our centers or other pain clinics is not likely to rid you, suddenly and magically, of all pain. But the opposite is equally true. Just because you have endured back pain for years, had one or more failed spinal surgeries, and have seen numerous specialists without help does not mean that you will not benefit from comprehensive interdisciplinary pain clinic intervention. In our program most sufferers can be helped but few will receive total and permanent relief. Whether you can be helped depends, in part, on realistic expectations.

Working to Quota

Physical exercise occupies a special and important place in the treatment of chronic back pain. Following an acute injury, most of us protect the injured body part in an effort to reduce the pain until the injured area has had time to heal. For example, if you have ever experienced an ankle sprain, you know that putting weight on the injured foot can cause considerable pain. Limping is the body's natural protection device to keep us from further harm until the ankle is healed. And if the injury is to the low back, we may, more guardedly and slowly, rotate the entire body rather than spontaneously turn and twist. Furthermore, because of the pivotal location and function of the lower back, almost any movement results in pain, so we sharply curtail our physical activities. Over time muscles that are no longer being used and exercised will contract and become weak. Physical conditioning deteriorates and the body becomes "tight." After months of decreased use, muscles become so contracted and weak that their use results in immediate discomfort. By this time the original cause of the pain may have healed or improved, yet severe pain on movement is still experienced. However, the pain may now be partially the result of weak and contracted muscles and tendons, rather than the original injury itself. Because pain on movement is experienced, we further restrict our motion and the cycle progresses from bad to worse.

For chronic back pain victims, physical exercise usually results in significant improvement in body tone and reduced pain. But perhaps you have tried to exercise and to be more physically active in the past only to find that your back pain increased and that you paid dearly for what later seemed to be an exercise mistake.

This is not uncommon and usually results from what is termed "working to tolerance." In other words, perhaps you overdid the exercise and activity and overextended your weakened muscles and body. Depending on how deconditioned you are, this can result from only minimal exercise.

In our treatment programs, we guard against the effects of "working to tolerance" by setting your physical reconditioning program on a "working-to-quota" basis. Working to quota simply means that we first find out how much activity you can tolerate *without* causing your back to hurt worse. If we use a stationary bicycle as an example, some back pain victims can pedal a mile, whereas others may be able to pedal only 100 feet before the activity causes increased back pain. Once we know your level (which is called your baseline), we schedule your exercise and activity program around this level. Suppose, for example, you can pedal 500 feet before your back pays the price. With 500 feet as your baseline, we would ask you to begin a daily routine of pedaling the stationary bicycle 475 feet. This, of course, does not increase your pain because the goal of 475 feet is below your baseline level. After several days of this routine, we would increase your quota of pedaling to perhaps 500 feet. But by the time your quota is raised, your body has gained enough strength to be able to accommodate this slight increase. As your body continues to grow stronger, your quota is increased gradually.

Over time most of our patients will build up their capacity for physical activity by an average of 343 percent. And by using the working-to-quota method, few patients experience any increase in the intensity of their back discomfort.

Modifying Your Pain Behavior

Even when your back pain lingers on and on, there are ways to make yourself feel better. In our programs we have found that the following hints work for many people. If you are a patient in one of our centers, professional staff members will work closely with you toward accomplishing the following:

1. *Realize that although others can try to help, only you can make yourself feel better.* Your doctor, family, and friends can give you advice and support, but you must assume responsibility for alleviating your pain and for taking an active role in the management of your pain problem. Chronic back pain is seldom a problem for a doctor to cure, but more frequently is a problem for you to manage.

2. *Gradually decrease the amount of medication you take.* Pain relievers rarely help chronic back pain. After you have taken a pain medication for a prolonged time, your body develops a tolerance, so the drug no longer provides relief. It may make you feel better, but this is because your body has become dependent on the medication. Due to this dependence, your doctors will not stop the medication abruptly. Instead we slowly reduce the amount of medication that you take, giving your body a chance to adapt to being without the drug. More will be said about drug detoxification in the following section.

3. *Focus on your activities rather than on your pain.* Try to stop thinking and talking about how much you hurt, as it will only make you feel worse. Remember the doctor when you were a child who advised you to look elsewhere when being given an injection because looking would cause the shot to hurt more? Attention to pain increases pain. Becoming more physically active and concentrating on alternatives will help take your mind off your pain.

4. *Gradually increase your level of activity.* Unless your doctor has a specific and sound reason to advise against it, physical activity is not harmful even with chronic back pain. Acute pain, such as that from a twisted ankle, is a protective and warning signal that rest is needed. However, when pain has continued for several months, its presence does not necessarily mean that something bad will happen if you gradually increase your level of physical

activity. As mentioned in the previous section, our programs utilize a successful working-to-quota system to increase physical activity.

5. *Go back to work.* Working is good for us, and especially good for chronic back pain victims. Working is an excellent example of "well behavior." Working provides a good reason to get up and get dressed each morning and will help you keep active and physically conditioned. With education and practice in pain control strategies, body mechanics, and other techniques discussed in this book, chronic back pain is seldom a totally disabling disorder.

Drug Detoxification

How many different medications have you tried to relieve your back discomfort? Two? Five? Ten? The fact is that most chronic pain patients have been extensively treated with multiple tranquilizers, sedatives, narcotics, and synthetic pain relievers, frequently leading to drug tolerance and dependence. Unfortunately not only do analgesic medications lose their effectiveness after several months, but they also cause personality changes and influence mental capabilities. Furthermore, they often decrease your ability to cope with pain and to think clearly. This may ultimately hinder efforts to return to a more normal and productive life-style.

In our programs one of our goals is to reduce—slowly, but steadily—drug dependence and consumption. This is called drug detoxification and has been effective in helping victims better manage their discomfort. We have had countless patients taking numerous medications for pain control report that they experienced significantly less pain following drug withdrawal than they suffered while taking drugs meant to reduce pain. The reason is simple. Analgesic drugs are designed and effective for short-term use with *acute* pain, not long-term use with *chronic* pain.

In our clinical programs, drug detoxification is accomplished by giving pain medications in a "pain cocktail"—a mixture of medications in a liquid form. The medication, masked with cherry syrup, is administered on a time-contingent basis rather than "as needed." In other words, you are given the pain cocktail every four hours rather than just when you feel it necessary. Over time the amount of active medication ingredients is gradually reduced to allow the body time to adjust to decreased medication intake. Seldom is a patient aware of the gradual reduction leading to ultimate elimination of medication, even when consumption has included numerous addicting drugs over a period of years. What is most often noticed is pain reduction!

Education

All treatments and therapies at our centers include education and present ways to apply what you have learned about controlling back pain. In addition to learning a number of specific pain control techniques, we believe that the more you know about the causes and effects of chronic pain, the better you will be able to manage your discomfort.

In our programs a pain group, led by a clinical psychologist, will meet with you and your family to discuss the social and personal issues involved in chronic pain, how it develops, and what is necessary to change the condition. You will also attend Pain School daily. Pain School is taught by various members of our staff and is designed to review such areas as basic anatomy and physiology, the differences between acute and chronic pain, the benefits of physical exercise, nutrition and weight control, back pain and sexual functioning, techniques for improved sleep, and coping with stress.

Body mechanics classes are also scheduled several times each week. These classes offer helpful guidance in correct posture, abdominal strengthening exercises, common proper and improper body movements, body technique for housework and vocational chores, the important role of muscles and back pain, and more. With proper use of the body, you will find that you hurt less and can engage in more physical activities. Education is a vital part of our rehabilitation philosophy of pain control.

PSYCHOLOGICAL REHABILITATION

Throughout this book we have emphasized the fact that chronic back pain is a biphasic or psychobiological disorder, composed of both physical and psychological components. *Do not allow this fact to threaten you!* We use the term "psychological" not to suggest that your back pain is "all in your head" nor that you are "crazy." Not at all. The psychological component of chronic back pain is completely normal. The body and mind simply cannot be separated and the effects of one will have direct effects on the other. For example, stress and tension (psychological) can result in stomach ulcers and headaches (physical). And recall our earlier discussion of the pain–tension cycle, and the fact that any chronic physical problem may result in frustration, irritation, anxiety, or depression (psychological) which compounds the problem and pain.

Given that the psychobiological nature of chronic back pain is normal, the smart victim of back pain will utilize this knowledge to achieve effective pain control. At our centers we can show you how.

Coping with Negative Feelings

How frequently do you awaken to the thought that the only things to look forward to that day are pain, irritation, disagreements with family or friends, pressures from bill collectors, frustration, embarrassment, depression, despair, and a host of other negative thoughts and feelings? Living with chronic back pain, 24 hours a day, 365 days a year, can gradually drain the strongest person of hope and optimism. There is little wonder that, in time, many intractable pain patients ask me, "Why should I even try to go on? This is not living—this is nothing more than existing in hell. If nothing can help, then I don't want to go on living."

It is easy to understand how chronic back pain victims can come to dwell on the negative, but this type of thinking is both unfortunate and unnecessary. Dr. David Bresler in his book *Free Yourself From Pain* warns pain victims to avoid identifying and *becoming* negative emotions. For example, see if you can detect the difference between reacting to an emotion in the following ways:

1. "I am depressed."
2. "There are feelings of depression passing through me."

In the first example, the negative emotion has actually become part of you and you, in turn, have become totally identified with it. In the second example, you perceive the emotion, but do not treat it as being intimately tied to your own life.

We attempt to help you learn to better cope with the negative feelings of helplessness and hopelessness that are so often associated with chronic back pain. We suggest that you treat yourself as you would treat your spouse, parent, or best friend. You would never encourage someone dear to you to think about how bad the past has been and how lousy the future will be. You would not tell that person to think about the pain and misery, and to concentrate on the negative but would encourage an emphasis on the positive. And if you would never say such negative things to someone else, then why say such things to yourself?

In our programs we do not allow negative thinking by either patients or staff. The atmosphere is positive, optimistic, and energetic. Retake control of your life and approach effective pain control with positive energy. The effect could change your life.

Behavior Modification

Remember our discussion in Chapters 1 and 3 of how long-term pain can become an unconscious habit? Researchers have repeatedly proved that with daily misery and pain comes a gradual expectancy to hurt, and with this expectancy often comes continued pain. This is conditioned or learned pain and can be thought of as "the bad habit of pain." This does not mean that you do not *really* hurt, but only that your body and mind are operating to "fuel the flame" of pain outside of your consciousness.

In our programs we utilize the principles of behavior modification to alter the bad habit of pain. One of the major differences between our treatment and an acute care treatment plan is that *all* of our therapies are designed to encourage well behaviors to and discourage pain behaviors. It will be requested that you avoid talking about your pain except at designated times, have your meals in the cafeteria, clean and straighten your own room, come to the nursing desk for medications, and participate in other strategies designed to promote independence and well behavior. In fact, in our programs you will be treated more as students or athletes in training than as traditional hospital patients. You will be expected to work hard and become actively involved in your pain management program.

Vocational Therapy

I am of the strong opinion that working is physically and psychologically beneficial for practically everyone, but particularly for the chronic back pain victim. But if you despise your job, that can create tension and stress, which may compound your pain problem. And if you are vocationally disabled due to back pain, the loss of income, self-worth, and self-concept and the financial strain may create even more stress and damaging tension.

Based on my training and experience in working with thousands of chronic back pain victims I believe that *chronic back pain is seldom a vocationally disabling problem*—an opinion that is guaranteed to elicit opposition from some health professionals and pain victims.

But if my reasoning is correct, why are hundreds of thousands of back pain victims registered as vocationally disabled on the rolls of Social Security disability, worker's compensation, and various social assistance programs? In my opinion this answer has two parts. The first is that these disabled pain victims have not had access to comprehensive interdisciplinary pain treatment centers where pain reduction and physical and psychological rehabilitation are emphasized. The second is that our system of Social Security and worker's compensation rewards and reinforces continued pain and disability while discouraging employment.

In our pain therapy programs, one of our major goals is to return back pain victims to suitable employment. In our experience back pain victims who are employed feel better; experience less pain, less depression, and less tension and anxiety; and enjoy a better self-concept.

The means by which we encourage suitable employment is vocational counseling and therapy. If you are working but are dissatisfied with your employment, our vocational counselor will explore alternatives. If you are unemployed, our vocational counselor will assess your career interests, talents, and capabilities. Perhaps you cannot work in a strenuous job such as loading trucks, but with proper body mechanics and adherence to the Tollison Program, most pain victims can perform some type of productive employment. This may also require job retraining or additional education, but seldom do graduates of our programs who have learned to manage their discomfort find that they can do "nothing" because of pain.

Vocational disability fosters feelings of helplessness, hopelessness, worthlessness, and stress that compound the multifaceted problems of chronic back pain.

Psychotherapy

If chronic back pain were isolated to body tissue injury, it would not be nearly the engulfing problem that it is. But your pain is not confined to your aching back alone. Chronic back pain affects practically every part of you—physically, mentally, socially, vocationally, and avocationally—and perception of pain is strongly influenced by psychological variables. Consider Farmer Brown who, while casually walking across a pasture, accidentally steps in a hole and sprains his ankle. He sits in the grass a long time in intense pain and then struggles to his feet and slowly hobbles toward the farmhouse. He hears an unnerving sound, immediately stops, and whirls around to see a huge bull charging toward him. Farmer Brown reacts instantly, running toward the fence and the safety of the other side with lightning quickness; the agony of the sprained ankle is forgotten in the overwhelming urgency of escaping the stampeding bull. When safely outside the fenced pasture and with the raging bull turned away, the ankle begins to throb and ache once again, and Farmer Brown agonizingly limps toward home.

In our programs we teach patients to use the most powerful pain control agent known—the human mind—to ease the multiple burdens of chronic back pain. In our daily group and individual therapy sessions, we teach you how to focus your concentration on topics other than pain and suffering, how to think more positive thoughts, how to avoid using pain as an escape, and how to manage stress in a positive manner. In our relaxation training classes, we teach you how to relax, how to enjoy improved rest and sleep, and how to reduce the anxiety and irritation so often closely related to chronic back pain. We also work with you to educate you in topics related to sexual functioning and improved communication.

At our PAIN THERAPY CENTERS℠, our patients learn in psychotherapy that they have two choices: either learn to control their pain, or allow their pain to control them.

Family Counseling

One of the many unique features of PAIN THERAPY CENTERS℠ programs is our belief in the importance of the family's role in effective pain management. Consider just a few of the many ways in which family members can influence your pain. Does your family reinforce your pain by paying attention to you only when you hurt? Does your family reinforce your pain by overly protecting you, "babying" you, and encouraging you to "take it easy?" Or maybe the other extreme is true. Is your family critical of you and your pain problem? Do frequent family arguments and disagreements create additional tension and stress in your life, which increases pain? Or is your family so uninvolved that the neutrality alone sabotages effective pain management? For example, does your family fail to encourage your compliance with the pain treatment program prescribed for you?

Just as there are many ways in which family members can sabotage effective pain control efforts, so too are there many ways in which they can be taught to serve as an ally in pain management. We regularly meet with family members of pain victims and teach them to be our treatment "extenders" once the patient returns home, frequently reviewing the goals of our program to reduce pain, reduce medication for pain relief, increase physical activity, and decrease the communication of pain. We recommend the following:

1. *Do not talk about pain.* Someone who talks about the pain is going to feel worse. Try these suggestions:
   a.   When your family member talks about the pain, try to divert his or her attention by introducing a new subject at the first opportunity.
   b.   When he or she talks about the pain, break eye contact.
   c.   Avoid asking about the pain. Instead, focus on his or her activities. For instance, when you return from work or shopping, don't ask how the person feels, but what he or she did while you were gone.
2. *Help your friend or relative increase his or her physical activity level. Activity is not harmful even when it hurts.* Only acute pain, such as that due to a strain or sprain, requires rest. After pain has continued for several months, the presence of pain upon movement usually means that the part is stiff and weak from lack of use. As the muscles get back into shape, the pain will probably diminish.
3. *As a family member of a chronic back pain victim, you can assist by doing the following:*
   a.   Give encouragement by praising increases in activity and when the person seems to be faltering.
   b.   Plan interesting activities both in and out of the home.
   c.   Avoid reinforcing or rewarding your family member by responding to complaints of pain.

Follow-up

Effective chronic pain management is a disciplined life-style and a lifetime program, not a short-term treatment program. To manage back discomfort successfully and return to a more productive life-style requires that you incorporate the principles and techniques described in this book and essentially "live" the Tollison Program.

To become lazy and drift away from the pain management program is almost certain to result in an increase in your pain and a return to misery, disability, irritation, and despair.

In PAIN THERAPY CENTERS℠ programs, we encourage patients to make follow-up visits once or twice monthly for a minimum of one year. When patients return they are involved in the same program in which they participated during their hospitalization. In this way our staff can encourage strict adherence to the management program, as well as address small problems that occasionally arise before they become more difficult problems. In our programs no charge is made for follow-up treatment and our research has indicated that patients who keep regular follow-up appointments experience less pain and make greater progress than patients who elect not to continue.

While chronic back pain may not be a totally curable problem, it can be successfully reduced and managed. As we have repeated throughout this book—either you can control your pain or allow it to control you!

16

A DAILY PLAN FOR PAIN MANAGEMENT: THE TOLLISON PROGRAM

As a youngster growing up in South Carolina, I knew two men who were involved in separate automobile accidents within a two-year period. They were about the same age, had similar jobs, lived within a mile or two of each other, had about the same level of education, and shared many other characteristics common to inhabitants of a small rural community. Both sustained injuries that required amputation of the left leg, just above the knee.

Although these men were alike in so many ways, there was one major factor that distinguished them—their life-styles following the accidents.

Frank had his doctor refer him to an area hospital for exhaustive, but helpful, rehabilitation training. He learned how to care for himself, to walk with a prosthesis, to be active and independent. He subsequently returned to work and his favorite hobby of fishing. I would see him at sporting events; he was the same Frank as before, only with a slight limp.

Ed was a different story. When he was released from the hospital, Ed went home and stayed there. He never worked again and was seen only when he made weekly visits to his doctor. Family members reported that Ed was practically helpless. He moved about the house in either a wheelchair or on crutches, needed assistance in dressing, and required that a family member care for his every need.

Frank and Ed shared such similar backgrounds and yet they had such vastly different reactions to their injuries. Why did Frank work hard to overcome his handicap while Ed essentially surrendered to his problems?

Years later, during my doctoral training, I treated hundreds of victims of pain and injury. Like Frank and Ed, some of them effectively controlled their pain whereas others allowed their pain to control them. While observing and working with these individuals, I began to formulate and test my own ideas about the important factors that differentiated the "Franks" and "Eds" of the world. Through a great deal of trial and error, I ultimately formulated five general factors that I feel distinguish the "winners" from the "losers" in the battle against chronic pain:

1. Education
2. Motivation
3. Determination
4. Treatment
5. Responsibility

Education refers to the proper training required to learn the specialized skills of pain control. The "Franks" recognize the need for specialized training and practice and accept the fact that pain management is a skill that is learned, like any other skill. The "Eds" think they know it all and refuse to learn. Rather than moving ahead to rehabilitation training and education, they are stuck like a stereo's needle on a record, playing over and over and over again misery, suffering, and pain.

Motivation is a human quality that influences decision making and goal attainment and plays a major part in effective pain management. Its role in differentiating successful from unsuccessful pain management can again be illustrated by my friends Frank and Ed. Frank made the decision to move on with his life and concentrate on his *abilities*. Ed made the decision (unconscious perhaps) that his life had essentially stopped at the time of the accident and concentrated on his *disabilities*.

Determination is a cognitive quality, possessed by many individuals, that ensures that they are not detoured or blocked from a desired goal. Some pain victims simply refuse to allow back pain to keep them from hobbies, work, or other priority activities; other victims find it impossible to stand up to their pain. The "winners" see pain as a formidable enemy they are determined to control; the "losers" submit to what they perceive as an insurmountable foe.

The need for medical *treatment* for back pain will vary depending on whether your pain is acute or chronic. Acute pain is discomfort of relatively recent onset that should be medically investigated, diagnosed, and treated. Chronic back pain is different and may persist for months, and even years, despite numerous diagnostic procedures and multiple treatments. In many cases of chronic back pain, the treatment goal is management rather than cure. Back pain winners accept this and avoid excessive overutilization of and dependency on our health-care system. Losers never accept this fact and sometimes spend years "doctor shopping," trying this and that drug, this surgery and that treatment, and always expecting a cure to be just around the corner at the next doctor's office.

Responsibility is perhaps the most important of the five differentiating factors and again is most relevant to victims of chronic back pain. When one lives with a chronically painful back, it is easy to cast the burden of responsibility for pain and suffering on others. Doctors are a prime target and I frequently hear it said, "If only I could find a competent doctor, I could get some relief from this pain." We have become a society of passive health-care recipients, eager to transfer the responsibility for our well-being to others. In all fairness it should be said that some doctors are partially to blame for encouraging this situation. And there are others to be blamed as well. The Eds of the world are quick to delegate responsibility for their aching backs to family members, employment situations, attorneys, Social Security disability, or worker's compensation insurance, whereas back pain winners accept the responsibility for the management of their pain, while utilizing the assistance of doctors, family, employers, attorneys, and society where appropriate.

These five factors—education, motivation, determination, treatment, and responsibility—spell the difference between effective and ineffective management of chronic back pain. If you want to be a back pain winner, this book is designed to help. The back care program presented is almost identical to that at the treatment centers that I founded and direct. Read the book a second time and make sure you have the entire program clear in your mind. And before starting your rehabilitation, discuss the program with your doctor and request his or her opinion.

When you are ready, begin your daily program of back pain management and practice, practice, practice! Do not become impatient. Effective pain management is a skill that takes time to learn and develop. Write the five factors that differentiate successful back pain management on an index card and place it on your dresser or bathroom mirror as a daily reminder. Progress will be slow but steady. Keep in mind that you are embarking on a *lifetime* program of pain management.

SOME HELPFUL HINTS

Distraction

If you need a bit of extra help, consider the following hints.

Concentration is a skill that can be developed with practice in much the same way that skills in golf, cooking, swimming, or playing tennis can be sharpened. Intense concentration on something other than pain will block the discomfort from your consciousness. Your mind, which can only fully concentrate on one thought or object at a time, will be distracted from the perception of pain. Dentists have long used distraction as a pain management technique by placing the dental chair so that the patient can look out a window or by hanging a picture on a wall in front of the patient. Distraction techniques that may work for you include mental arithmetic problems such as counting backward by threes from 100, or even sexual fantasies!

Stopping Negative Self-Talk

Most of us spend a good part of every day "talking to ourselves." Silent internal dialog, or self-talk, is a way of planning and organizing our thoughts and feelings. Since pain is a negative sensation, our self-talk about thoughts and feelings of pain is also usually negative. Negative self-talk is associated with anxiety and increased pain. It has not occurred to most people that internal statements, or self-talk, can be managed and controlled with practice, thereby reducing discomfort and pain.

Positive Thinking

A change from negative self-talk to positive thinking can have a significant effect on the pain you experience. Just as negative self-talk is associated with anxiety and increased pain, positive thinking is associated with and reinforces confidence, relaxation, and equanimity. It requires determination and practice, but the results can be a dramatic reduction in back pain intensity.

Controlling Anxiety

It has been noted throughout this text that anxiety and associated muscle tension increase pain levels, while relaxation and calm are associated with decreased pain intensity. Mental and physiological calm are required for effective pain control. To control anxiety practice the progressive relaxation exercises outlined in Chapter 10 until you can achieve a state of deep muscular and mental relaxation within minutes. In addition, try wearing a rubber band around your wrist as a reminder to pause periodically throughout the day, slowly count backward from ten to zero, take a deep breath, and relax!

Concentrating on Abilities, Not Disabilities

One of the many complexities associated with chronic back pain is that patients naturally focus on activities that were once a part of their lives, and now believe impossible because of pain. Such activities may include recreational and vocational interests. Understandably, many chronic back pain patients concentrate on activities in which they can no longer participate, and pain becomes the center of their lives. To avoid the increased pain and misery such thinking creates, spend time identifying and perfecting your abilities. If you can no longer play football, how about softball? If you can no longer perform a job that requires sitting eight hours each day, how about one that involves walking? Chronic back pain is *not* a totally disabling disorder. Some concentration on your abilities, rather than your disabilities, will prove this to be true!

TO CONCLUDE

With the five factors of success clearly in mind, a few extra hints for those particularly tough days, a great deal of patience, and the

Tollison Program to follow, you too can become a winner in the daily battle against chronic back pain. I hope you accept the challenge.

I wish you much success!

Appendix A

THE MOST FREQUENTLY ASKED QUESTIONS ABOUT BACK PAIN

At our PAIN THERAPY CENTERS™ programs, we see hundreds of back pain victims each year. And almost every back pain victim has a question or two about his or her aching back. Here are some of the most frequently asked questions and my responses.

1. Q—I injured my back two months ago in an automobile accident. Since that time I have been told by two different doctors to stay in bed as much as possible and to take it easy until the pain goes away. Then you tell me to become involved in a supervised exercise program. Who is right?

A—The answer depends on the type of injury you sustained, the presence of any complicating medical disorders, and a host of other variables. But in a general sense, the argument of bed rest versus activity is a philosophical difference of opinion among health care professionals.

The "bed rest" group believes that taking to bed and reducing physical activity constitute the treatment of choice for back pain, particularly acute or recent back discomfort. This thinking has long been taught in schools of medicine and many doctors accept it without question.

The "exercise and activity" group believes that a day or two of bed rest is permissible, but that additional inactivity may prolong recovery following most back injuries or episodes of increased pain. This group generally believes that the sooner you start a specialized and supervised program of back-strengthening exercises and return to regular activities, the faster your back will respond with reduced pain. The "exercise and activity" group points out that women having babies, patients having surgery, and people suffering heart attacks were once told to stay in bed for days, weeks, and sometimes months. But because of additional information, we now know that women having babies and patients having surgery, whenever possible, should be out of bed and walking within hours of the procedure. And patients suffering a heart attack are likely to be enrolled in a cardiac rehabilitation program with strenuous physical exercise within a week or two of the attack. Proponents of the "exercise and activity" philosophy of back pain treatment believe that supervised and special exercise promotes healing and functioning, and there is a steadily increasing amount of scientific research to bolster their argument.

2. Q—My doctor once told me that if I lost 40 pounds my back would feel better. Do you agree?

   A—If you are obese, there is little question that losing weight will reduce the weight and strain on your back. Obesity seldom *causes* back pain but can certainly complicate an existing back problem. Think of your body weight and back like this: If you put the motor from a small compact automobile into a large luxury limousine, the motor will be required to work extra hard to pull the heavy weight. On the other hand, putting the motor from a large limousine into a compact car will place little demand on the motor.

   Obesity places extra work on the spine and your back must work harder to support you. An already aching back will likely protest. Losing weight reduces the workload on the back.

   But losing weight alone is seldom enough to make a major difference in the amount of pain you suffer. Strengthening the back and abdominal muscles, using proper body mechanics, and practicing the other components of back care described in this book will offer you the best chance for back pain relief.

3. Q—My doctor says that I have myofascial back pain. What does this mean?

   A—Myofascial simply means "muscle" or soft tissue. What your doctor was probably trying to explain is that your back discomfort is caused by muscle and soft tissue, such as a muscle strain. And don't be too quick to discount the seriousness of muscle strain or the amount of back pain that can result from it. Probably more chronic back pain results, at least in part, from muscle strain than from any other single cause. And because of the pivotal location of the spinal musculature, repeated poor body mechanics, deconditioned life-styles, obesity, and a host of other variables, the pain of a back strain can cause months, and even years, of suffering. Most experts agree that a proper program of instruction and body mechanics and spinal care combined with a graduated and supervised program of strengthening exercises, as soon as possible after an acute muscle strain injury, can usually resolve the problem much faster than bed rest, and return you to normal functioning with less pain.

4. Q—A friend tells me that a back brace will ease my pain. She has been wearing one for several months and claims that her back causes only minimal problems as long as she wears the brace. What do you think?

A—First, you should discuss this with your doctor before purchasing a brace or corset. Your personal physician is in the best position to advise you about the advantages and disadvantages of bracing in your particular situation.

Back braces were once frequently employed in the treatment of back misery. And for good reason—back pain victims reported less pain when wearing a brace. The reason is simple. Most back braces are sturdy enough to perform the work of holding you upright and supporting the spine. When a brace performs this job, the back doesn't have to work. Many people report almost instant relief, at least as long as they wear the brace.

But if the back is not allowed to exercise and do its job, it soon becomes weak and lazy. In time the braced back may become so weak and deconditioned that it can no longer perform its duties without help from the brace. Your back is then dependent on the brace for help and, rather than your back becoming stronger and resisting further injury or damage, it becomes weaker and more susceptible to future injury, and you are forced to wear the brace almost constantly.

Many experts believe that a back brace is occasionally permissible for a few days at a time, but caution should be used to avoid making a bad situation worse!

5. Q—My back pain is not severe, but has gradually increased in intensity. I think that I should see a doctor. But who—family doctor, orthopedic surgeon, neurosurgeon, member of a pain clinic, chiropractor? Why are so many doctors involved with the back, and where do I start?

A—It is true that a variety of specialists lay claim to the painful back, and this can be confusing. Part of the reason for this is that the volume of medical information has forced doctors to specialize in limited areas in order to keep up with all that is new and constantly changing. A second reason is that a painful human spine is so complicated that the knowledge required to address the problem spills over into a variety of medical specialties. To answer your question, let us quickly review those specialists who most frequently work with painful backs.

A *family physician* usually knows you and your family well. He or she knows about the kidney trouble that you had last year, the fall off the horse you had as a child, the sore throat and cough you suffered last Christmas, what medications work well for you, and the drugs to which you are allergic, as well as that your mother died of cancer, and that you sometimes have tension headaches when your job is particularly stressful. The family physician not only knows you and your family, but sees you as a "whole" person rather than as specialized parts.

The *orthopedic surgeon* is a specialist in the bones and joints of your body and is well trained to correct certain body problems surgically. Since the back is partially composed of bones and joints, frequently the orthopedic suregeon will be consulted to determine if surgery to those bones and joints is needed to correct your back problem.

The *neurosurgeon* is a specialist in the brain, nerves, and nervous systems of the body. Since the back has numerous nerves that enter and exit the spine, a neurosurgeon may be consulted to determine if surgery is needed to correct a problem with one or more of the spinal nerves.

Most *pain clinics* do not serve as diagnostic facilities to determine why your back is hurting, but rather provide specialized nonsurgical treatment to reduce back misery. Pain clinics deal more with the pain itself, not the cause of pain.

Chiropractors are specialists in spinal anatomy and non-surgical manipulation of the spine. While there are differing schools of chiropractic philosophy, most chiropractors combine spinal manipulation with physical treatments, such as ultrasound and heat, in an attempt to reduce certain types of back pain.

As you can probably see, the family physician is in the best position to "quarterback" both the diagnosis and treatment of your back misery. The family physician may refer you to the various specialists mentioned, but can best compile the various pieces of information and correctly counsel you.

6. Q—What about the use of muscle relaxant medications in treating back pain?

A—I have two major problems with the use of muscle relaxant medications. The first is that muscle relaxants do not cure back misery but only temporarily mask the symptoms. I'm often reminded of a patient I treated years ago for alcoholism. He maintained that he drank alcohol (a drug) to escape the misery of his life (symptoms). But when he became sober, the misery of his life was still there (symptoms) and he also had a terrible headache. Rather than dealing with the real cause of his misery, he would attempt to mask the symptoms again by consuming more alcohol. Taking muscle relaxants is often the same. Rather than taking action to eliminate or control the cause of back pain, many individuals and doctors elect to use muscle relaxants to disguise the symptoms temporarily. When the effects of the medication wear off, the back misery is still there. And then what? Take more medication?

The second problem is that it often leaves you feeling sleepy, drugged, groggy, and generally quite miserable. This is because muscle relaxant medication is nonselective. Muscle relaxants don't work just on the muscles in the back, but on muscles throughout your body. It's an all-or-nothing type of phenomenon and the result generally is that the individual is too groggy to work to remedy the back problem.

7. Q—My doctor sounds like a broken record. Every time I tell him my back hurts, he starts talking about my posture. What's so important about posture?

A—Obviously a great deal more than either you know or are willing to accept. Body posture can have a great effect on the body, and particularly the back. For example, if you don't have back problems, improper body posture can set the stage for back injury or the gradual onset of back pain. And if your back is already painful, improper body posture can be the cause of your discomfort, or serve as a contributing factor in your pain.

The human body is structured in a balanced symmetrical design that is truly a mechanical marvel. The body functions through the use of pulleys and levers and is balanced both left and right, as well as top and bottom. It may come as a surprise to you to learn that the structure and function of the human body have served as a model and catalyst for the design of countless everyday machines and equipment.

Interfere with the balance of the body and its levers and pulleys through faulty posture and you can usually expect trouble. Not only do you crowd internal organs, but often you place excessive weight and wear on the spine. The result can be back pain. Listen to your doctor. Since improper posture is usually the result of habit, practice proper posturing and see if your back problem doesn't improve.

8. Q—I tried some of the exercises that you propose and found that I experienced increased pain. Do I stop or keep going?

   A—If you have properly performed the exercises that I have included in this book and find that you hurt more, you should stop exercising until you can discuss this with your doctor. However, you should make certain that you are performing the exercises correctly. The exercise program outlined here is intended to be started slowly and gradually, after your doctor's approval. Do not become impatient and attempt too much, too quickly! Carefully read the section on "working to quota" and do not exceed your quotas, even if you feel you can. Be consistent. Exercise every day rather than sporadically.

   It is also important that you fully realize the important difference between *pain* and *damage*. The exercise program outlined may cause you a week or so of mildly increased general muscle soreness. This is so because you are using muscles that, perhaps, you haven't exercised in some time. But the exercises should not cause damage to your back if you obtain your doctor's approval prior to beginning and implement the exercise program as outlined.

9. Q—It seems that my back has hurt for so long that I'm now becoming depressed. Is this normal?

   A—Not only it is perfectly normal, but it would be abnormal if you suffered months or years of back misery and did *not* become depressed! It is important to realize that pain is more than a physical perception. Pain has at least two major components—physical and psychological. Acute or short-term pain is usually associated with anxiety. If you slam an automobile door on a finger, not only will you hurt, but your heart rate increases, your blood pressure soars, adrenalin is released in your body, and you become agitated, frightened, and anxious.

Chronic, or long-term, pain is different. Chronic pain is most associated with depression. If your finger injured from the automobile door accident continues throbbing and aching months after the injury, you are likely to become depressed. This is so because of the gradual wearing on your emotional state, your altered life-style and altered concentration. Again, this is a normal reaction to suffering chronic pain. And in time the physical and psychological components can become so interrelated that the physical pain is intensifying the psychological depression, and the psychological depression is intensifying the pain. Although this situation is not abnormal, it can create intense and prolonged suffering for back pain victims. Our programs recognize the biphasic composition of chronic back pain and target treatment toward both the physical and psychological components of pain in order to return the pain sufferer to a more normal and productive life.

10. Q—In 25 words or less, tell me how to reduce my back pain.
    A—Exercise, relax, use ice massage, avoid medications when possible, avoid surgery unless truly indicated, accept the responsibility for your back, reread this book, and *practice!*

INDEX